What This Book Is About . . .

- This book shows you how to revolutionize your health and well-being by using a simple, safe, and effective means of bowel cleansing.

- This book explains how the underactive condition of your elimination organs influences the development of illness and disease in your body.

- This book reveals the intimate connection between the bowel and internal organs in the development of the embryo and how this connection determines future disease and dysfunction in the body.

- This books describes the role of the neural-arc reflex in the generation of disease and what you can do about it.

- This book presents the amazing Ultimate Tissue Cleansing Program for cleansing the bowel directly and other tissues indirectly.

- This book contains a wealth of practical ideas on how to improve your lifestyle, nutrition, personal habits, and thinking in order to work your way toward better health.

DR. JENSEN'S GUIDE TO BETTER BOWEL CARE

DR. BERNARD JENSEN

AVERY
a member of Penguin Putnam Inc.

The therapeutic procedures in this book are based on the training, personal experiences, and research of the author. Because each person and situation are unique, the author and publisher urge the reader to check with a qualified health professional before using any procedure when there is any question regarding appropriateness.

The publisher does not advocate the use of any particular diet or health program, but believes the information presented in this book should be available to the public.

Because there is always some risk involved, the author and publisher are not responsible for any adverse effects or consequences resulting from the use of any of the suggestions, preparations, or procedures described in this book. Please do not use the book if you are unwilling to assume the risk. Feel free to consult with a physician or other qualified health professional. It is a sign of wisdom, not cowardice, to seek a second or third opinion.

Cover designer: Doug Brooks
In-house editor: Elaine Will Sparber
Typesetters: Helen Contoudis
    and Gary Rosenberg

Avery
a member of
Penguin Putnam Inc.
375 Hudson Street
New York, NY 10014
www.penguinputnam.com

Library of Congress Cataloging-in-Publishing Data
Jensen, Bernard, 1908–
    [Guide to better bowel care]
    Dr. Jensen's guide to better bowel care : a complete program for
tissue cleansing through bowel management / Bernard Jensen.
        p.   cm.
    Includes bibliographical references and index.
    ISBN 0-89529-584-9
    1. Intestines—Diseases. 2. Intestines—Care and hygiene.
    3. Constipation—Prevention.   I. Title.
    RC860.J46   1999
    616.3′4—dc21   98-22436
                                                                            CIP

Printed in the United States of America.

Contents

Contents

Acknowledgments

The quote on pages 31 to 32 is from Karl J. Isselbacher, et al. editors, *Harrison's Principles of Internal Medicine* © 1994 by The McGraw-Hill Companies. Reproduced with the permission of The McGraw-Hill Companies.

I must give foremost credit to Sir Arbuthnot Lane, physician to the British Royal Family, for helping me realize the relationship between the bowel and disease elsewhere in the body. Max Gerson, M.D., opened my eyes to the value of bowel cleansing in ridding the body of chronic and degenerative disease conditions. He proved it could be done. I appreciate John Harvey Kellogg, M.D., of Battle Creek, Michigan, for teaching me the importance of proper bowel flora. I have Drs. Denis P. Burkett and Neil D. Painter to thank for their writings on the importance of dietary fiber, not only to improve bowel health and quicken bowel transit time, but to reduce the incidence of bowel-related diseases elsewhere in the body. I am grateful to the homeopathic physician Constantine Hering for formulating a law of cure that emphasizes that healing takes place "from the inside out."

I would like to thank William Welles, D.C., for his contributions and research concerning bowel health and proper elimination. Alan Immerman, D.C., has also graciously allowed me to use some of his bowel research. My relationship with Dr. V.E. Irons in bowel-care work goes back many years.

Donald Bodeen, D.C., and his wife, Joyce, made important contributions to this book. Joyce has conducted tissue-cleansing programs on the East Coast. My long-time girl Friday, Sylvia Bell, has helped in many of the tissue-cleansing programs here on the Ranch.

As always, deep appreciation goes to Marie Jensen, my wife, for her faithful support in all my work.

The quote on pages 31 to 32 is from Kurt J. Isselbacher, et al., editors, *Harrison's Principles of Internal Medicine*, © 1994 by The McGraw-Hill Companies. Reproduced with the permission of The McGraw-Hill Companies.

The original illustrations on pages 113, 114, 123, 124, and 128 are by John Wincek.

The illustrations on pages 150, 152, and 153 are used courtesy of Dr. William Welles.

The table on pages 157 to 159 is from E. Lanza and R.R. Butron: "A Critical Review of Food Fiber Analysis and Data." © 1986 by The American Dietetic Association. Reprinted by permission from the *Journal of the American Dietetic Association*, Volume 86 (1986), page 732.

The photographs on pages 213 to 222 were taken by Dr. Bernard Jensen.

Preface

My father was a chiropractor. I, too, sought to be a chiropractor, for I knew from my observations that this system of carefully examining and adjusting the spinal vertebrae produces results. Painful conditions are alleviated. Sick people get well, the lame walk, and the bent-over are able to again stand erect.

Upon graduation from chiropractic school, I was anxious to open my office. It wasn't long before I developed a busy practice. But I soon came to see that something was missing in my work. Although most of my colleagues were satisfied with their office practices, I was becoming increasingly dissatisfied. I noticed that the great majority of people who came to my office seemed to be content with the relief I was able to afford them with spinal adjustments, but that many continually came back with the same conditions. I was administering adjustments to their spines, but I discovered that what these people really needed more than anything were adjustments in their ways of living.

I began to see that people needed to be taught how to improve their lifestyles. Some were in need of mental and spiritual uplifts. Conditions in their lives had pulled them down, driven them to a state of negativity and despair. Some had jobs or careers for which they were physically or mentally ill-suited. Chronic stress and tension had become a way of life for them. Nearly all were in need of adjustments in their diets. Some didn't have time to eat correctly. They were always in a rush. Most, however, had the time to eat incorrectly, consuming foods prepared according to culinary habits passed down in their families. Nearly all lacked the knowledge of what constituted a health-sustaining diet, much less a health-building one. They were prime candidates for an educational adjustment.

I saw that for a lack of knowing a better way and without the benefit of proper guidance, my patients persisted in the ignorance that promotes chronic ill health. Although I was effecting wonderful relief through chiropractic adjustments, this therapy alone was often not enough to provide long-term changes. Dissatisfied and convinced that neither my patients nor I should continue in this situation, I became determined to make a change.

I opened my first sanitarium in Altadena, California, in the mountains, a spot considered by city dwellers at the time to be "out in the country." It had clean air and lots of sunshine, essential elements for health. There, I could finally monitor my patients and give them the education they needed to make changes in their lives, an education that was impossible to offer in an office practice. It worked, too!

In subsequent years, I moved to a larger facility. My largest sanitarium was the two-hundred-acre Hidden Valley Ranch in the mountains east of Escondido, California. There, I had everything I needed to help people find the path to health. People from all over the world came to stay for a while to learn the lessons of health, and the sanitarium eventually became quite famous.

Through the years, many different views of bowel care have been presented, creating some confusion about exactly what constitutes proper bowel hygiene. In this book, I give you the most complete information currently available and the wisdom accumulated over a lifetime devoted to natural therapeutics. This book is offered with the understanding that an individual can learn what is necessary for proper bowel management and to show the results that can be obtained by taking care of the bowel properly. No doctor should be without this knowledge. No doctor should practice any system of healing without first considering the five main elimination channels—the bowel, skin, kidneys, lymphatic system, and lungs—the most important of which is the bowel.

The response to the first edition of this book has been wonderful. I have received many suggestions and comments that have prompted me to revise and expand the book to make it more responsive to your needs. I have had many wonderful testimonials from people who successfully applied the lessons of this book!

The following pages give valuable information about the waste-elimination process, focusing on the bowel in particular. I have always made it a practice to check the main elimination channels on a patient's first visit to my office. Attempting to take care of any symptom in the body without a good elimination system is futile.

I have traveled to the farthest corners of the earth searching for the secrets to health and long life. I want to share my discoveries with you so that you, too, can partake of the increased well-being and enjoyment of life that can result. This book should awaken you to the realization that the greatest healing power comes from within. To this end, I am offering the insights and wisdom I've gathered over more than six decades of work in the healing arts and restoration of normal bowel function. In order for you to understand my work, I present a smattering of the anatomy and physiology of the digestive and elimination systems in Chapter 1. In Chapter 2, I discuss how digestive malfunction can cause toxins to build up in the intestines, which in turn can make the entire body ill. In Chapter 3, I discuss the bowel disorders that affect so many people that they are today considered common; and in Chapter 4, I explain how a problem in the bowel can cause symptoms in a seemingly unrelated part of the body. The heart and soul of this book are in Chapters 5 and 6, which together present my Ultimate Tissue Cleansing Program. The Seven-Day Cleansing Program, the first phase of the two-part program, is fully explained in Chapter 5; and the Seven-Week Building and Replacement Program, the second of the two phases, is detailed in Chapter 6. In Chapter 7, I outline the nutritional sins and dietary laws that form the base of my cleansing program, as well as my dietary and health beliefs in general. And finally, in Chapter 8, I present a few other dietary techniques for bowel management. This last chapter will be of special interest to those persons who wish to cleanse their bowel, but cannot at this point in their lives devote themselves to the full undertaking.

It often takes an act of resolution and courage to combat the bowel difficulties that so many people experience. There is no better way of resolving these difficulties than by taking positive action. The instructions given in this book will give you the opportunity to take greater responsibility for your level of health and well-being.

Introduction

How did I ever become involved with the bowel? The bowel was the last thing I wanted to focus on. It was the last thing that came to my mind. I used to think that when the bowel didn't work well, we should turn to a laxative. I didn't know there was a lifestyle that produces a healthy body. Today, I have found lifestyle to be the most important thing in the world.

As my attention turned increasingly toward the bowel, I began to look at the deaths of our political leaders and other great people with new eyes. All these people seemed to have complications. Every one of them seemed to have some disorder of the elimination system that contributed to his or her death. Take Frank Sinatra, for example. Mr. Sinatra went to the hospital with the symptoms of a heart attack and ended up with pneumonia. I firmly believe that he would not have come down with pneumonia if he didn't have an undetected bowel problem. The body is a community of many organs working for the good of one another. Without properly functioning elimination organs, the body dies.

The body is an organization. It digests food, processes oxygen, and undertakes numerous other activities. Every organ contributes something to the body and its activities. As human beings, we need every cell, tissue, and organ that was put into our body. The body is the instrument through which we live, and we should treat it with respect. We cannot take our body, so wonderfully put together, and expect it to function properly if we violate all the natural laws that are necessary for it to be well.

The first natural law is to feed the body natural food. We are meant to have fiber. We are meant to have natural enzymes. We are meant to have food in its raw state. When we begin to obey the natural laws again, it is almost like re-entering the Garden of Eden.

When we return to the Garden of Eden, consuming natural foods and following a more natural way of living, the bowel always responds. I've been told by patients so many times, "I am having natural bowel movements for the first time in twenty years." Some patients also tell me, "I am even having diarrhea. I am having a bowel movement every day instead of once every ten days." These patients mistake a return to regularity for diarrhea!

Most people don't understand the bowel. They don't know how to take care of it or how to meet its needs. We go through life violating the natural laws until we reach the point where the most natural thing left is our nutritional program and even that causes abuse to the bowel.

When the bowel is not taken care of, its responses become sluggish and underactive. It is not able to heal itself and does not have the ability to perform the things it was meant to do.

Food should pass through the body every eighteen hours. Any food that spoils, ferments, forms gas, or causes a disturbance in the bowel also affects the rest of the body. Above all things, it is necessary to have proper bowel movements in order to have a healthy body.

I realized early on in my practice that the bowel has to be taken care of. I started seriously caring for the bowel when I realized the good that an enema can do. I saw what a cleansing can do, and I think that I have probably been the most influential voice promoting the cleansing of the bowel. In fact, every patient I have ever treated with bowel cleansing has improved. Note that I did not say "was cured." Some did leave their health problems completely behind, but not all did. This is truly something to think about.

In the 1950s, I spent time with Dr. Max Gerson at his sanitarium in New Jersey. People at the time were crying out for medications in order to get relief from their various disorders. Max, an early proponent of bowel cleansing, said, "No, you need an enema, not a drug." Invariably, Max's enemas brought relief. Since he often administered enemas day and night to keep his patients' bowels as clean as possible, he had good success even with degenerative conditions. His book, *Fifty Cancer Patients Cured*, caused a significant stir in the medical community.

Is it a matter of treating disease? Are we treating the body? No, we are upgrading the ability of the bowel to work better. Are we cleaning out toxic material? Yes, because we have to.

I have always admired and believed in the work of John Tilden,

M.D. Dr. Tilden discovered that toxemia is at the root of most health problems and diseases. (For a full discussion of toxemia, see Chapter 2.) He wrote a book entitled *Toxemia Explained* that made quite an impact at the time of its publication. Dr. Tilden was widely respected, but his work has since been forgotten and neglected.

People demand relief from pain and discomfort. Their primary concern is temporary relief, not taking care of the problem at the root of their symptoms. What do we look back to as a cause?

Toxemia Explained is a book that everybody should have. No doctor should practice without it. I didn't always believe the bowel had to be taken care of first. But then I read another book, *Pandora's Box: What to Eat and Why* by J. Oswald Empringham. This book is about taking care of the bowel.

I also read with great interest the work of Sir W. Arbuthnot Lane, physician to the British Royal Family in the late nineteenth century and first half of the twentieth century. Dr. Lane was a master surgeon. One day, he operated on the bowel of an arthritic fourteen-year-old boy. After the surgery, the boy's arthritis was gone. This made Dr. Lane stop and think. Another of Dr. Lane's patients, a female, had a toxic thyroid gland. When he operated on the woman's bowel, her thyroid gland became normal. After many such experiences, Dr. Lane switched from practicing medicine to teaching nutrition and bowel care. During the final twenty-five years of his life, he brought out the fact that the bowel is the most important organ in the body to care for. What a wonderful discovery!

Dr. Lane's experience had a great influence on me. I said to myself, "Look again here. If there is a problem in the body and you take care of the bowel, every other organ will respond to it."

If waste cannot be eliminated and accumulates in the body, perhaps suppressed by drugs or extreme tiredness and fatigue, disease walks in. Bacteria accumulates. Worms and germ life develop most often in an underactive bowel. This is a big problem today. Gastrointestinal specialists realize that sulfa drugs and antibiotics destroy all bacteria—the friendly bacteria as well as the bad—in the bowel.

Much has been said by pediatricians about colostrum, the yellow fluid that precedes breastmilk, as the means of getting a new baby's bowel to function properly. This is most important. The first four days of a child's life are vital in getting the bowel off to a good start. Many new mothers don't realize this. They feed their babies formula. They try to replace a normal and natural substance with a factory-made concoction. More and more today, we are seeing the foolishness in this. Nature knows best, but sometimes humans have to find this out the hard way.

In my work, I often have to rehabilitate people and change their minds. Among my greatest experiences was seeing my children learn to take care of their bowel movements the right way. That is, I taught my children that they shouldn't "hold it." Holding back bowel movements is what causes diverticula (bowel pockets) to form in the lower segment of the colon. I taught my children that when their dog scratched at the screen door, it meant that he wanted to go out. I told them he was trying to say, "Let me out! I need to have a bowel movement!" Their canary, I showed them, had bowel movements right in its cage, no inhibitions whatsoever. But humans are foolish and often don't attend to their urges to have bowel movements. Today, people neglect their bowels as a matter of habit, and it's this neglect that I try to combat in my teachings and writings.

There is so much to learn about the bowel if you are willing to read books on the subject. You would be interested in what William Welles has done, and in what V.E. Irons has done. You would be interested in my visits to Battle Creek Sanitarium, where I went to find out what John Harvey Kellogg had to say about the bowel. Dr. Kellogg developed a method of changing the intestinal flora when it's not in balance. While I was visiting him, he came up with a culture that he sent to Dr. Allan Roy DaFoe, the doctor in Canada who was taking care of the Dionne quintuplets. Dr. DaFoe had telephoned Dr. Kellogg and said that he would probably lose one or two of the quints if he couldn't activate their bowels. Dr. Kellogg immediately sent an acidophilus culture to him. A couple of weeks later, Dr. DaFoe reported, "I believe we have saved the life of those infants by taking care of the bowel."

The rest of the bowel story is a more practical story. V.E. Irons made it practical. Kay Shaffer made it practical. I saw much of the work these two individuals did. Dr. Irons and Ms. Shaffer also worked with nutrition. They helped me see why Dr. V.G. Rocine pushed me into studying proper nutrition for the bowel and for the other parts of the body. Dr. Rocine believed that we can transcend our problems and develop a well body if we take care of our nutrition.

We have to consider diet when we are trying to improve our health. Health is not just a matter of taking an enema. It's also learning how to live in a healthy style. I believe that my nutritional teachings are among the finest available. Proper nutrition is what I use to rehabilitate people who have gone down the path of bad habits, including bad bowel habits. All nutrition affects the bowel. To find health by improving your nutrition but not using colemas or other bowel care is possible, although it's difficult.

But you know, there is one thing about using nutrition and natural cures to improve health, and this is the fact that they take too long to bring results. I tell my patients even to this day that it will take a year for their health problems to be solved and their bodies to become well again. It takes time—as much as seven years, they say—to make new bones. It takes just forty-eight hours to build new skin on the palm of the hand, but months to build a new stomach wall. It takes months to renew a kidney. So, we need to be patient while the body rebuilds and renews itself.

It would be convenient if a form of analysis existed for determining inherent weaknesses and toxic deposits in tissues. Colonic technicians cleanse the bowel, but many times they don't know the condition of the bowel or the composition of the bowel wall. They don't know its weaknesses or where toxic material has settled. They work blind, so to speak.

Despite this, in most cases colonic treatment brings good results. It would be better if we had a greater knowledge of the bowel, and not only of what is in the bowel, but of what toxic materials have been absorbed into the blood or lymph, and carried to other inherently weak organs in the body. When this happens, it is a form of suppression. We tend to blame medications for suppressing diseases and not allowing proper elimination to take place. But lifestyle can be a form of suppression. An imbalanced diet can be a form of suppression.

We shouldn't have to use laxatives to take care of the bowel. Many people are dependent upon laxatives. Roughly 18,000 tons of laxatives are sold in the United States every year. This is a lot of constipation and bowel troubles, friends, and it should tell us that we can't blame our problems only on our bowels. We need to look at our lifestyle habits and nutrition. We need to make changes. I learned a good deal about this from V.E. Irons, and from Kay Shaffer, who gave me my first colema. From my personal experience with bowel cleansing, I could see that I could do much good for my patients by introducing them to colemas. It was at this point that I started developing my own system for taking colemas.

Chronic diseases build up over long periods of time. About 80 percent of the patients who go to doctors have chronic diseases. The American Cancer Society says it takes twenty years to develop cancer. What are you developing in your bowel today? Do you know? Long before we notice any disease symptoms developing, we go blindly along, ignorant of what trouble may be developing in our bowel. We should do better than that. We should follow a preventive program.

I believe people need to be educated about prevention. Doctors can physically locate diverticula and gas by percussing (tapping) the bowel. They then know if the patient does or doesn't need bowel cleansing. Wherever diverticula are, a lot of putrifaction and fermentation are taking place. These are what caused the gas. These are what need to be eliminated from the bowel.

The bowel must be considered first in the disease-reversal process, according to Hering's Law of Cure. Constantine Hering was a homeopath who established the first school of homeopathy in the United States, in Philadelphia. His law, however, was never well received because it was never well understood. According to Hering's Law of Cure, "All cure starts from within out, from the head down, and in the reverse order as the symptoms appeared." It refers to the source of disease being in the bowel. As we take care of the bowel, we cleanse and purify the body and all its organs. That cleansing and purifying must start with the bowel.

Of course, we also have to consider the cleansing process in connection to the other four elimination channels—the skin, kidneys, lymphatic system, and lungs. The liver also needs to be in good working order because it is a detoxification organ. We have to make sure we have enough red blood cells. An anemic body doesn't have enough energy and doesn't eliminate well.

The whole body has to be put in order. But we must always start with cleansing and making sure that there are no toxic materials being absorbed from the bowel and settling in other organs. Doctors of late have been concerned with leaky bowel syndrome. When the bowel is underactive and constipated, whether it has diverticula or not, more toxins, cholesterol, and fats are leaked (forced) into the bloodstream and lymph. This is why we must speed up our bowel transit time, first by cleansing the bowel, then by consuming more high-fiber foods such as fruits, vegetables, legumes, and whole cereal grains.

The kidneys are taken care of as the bowel is cleansed. But even so, we must be careful not to give the kidneys too much to do, since if they are inherently weak, they will have problems. The consequences could include swollen ankles and increased blood urea and creatinine. These symptoms should vanish as the bowel becomes cleaner, however.

Doctors today can prevent many deaths by taking care of the bowel first. We have the technology. We have the knowledge. When will doctors open their eyes and see that there is a solution for the 80 percent of patients who have chronic diseases? The common bowel disorders also develop over a period of many years. Many begin with a stomachache. Sometimes an over-the-counter medication is taken to get rid of gas, for instance. Without correcting the diet producing the gas, however, we are playing with our future health. All chronic diseases arise out of neglect of beginning problems.

The other day I had a patient who said, "I would like you to take care of me. How can I get well?" The first thing I noticed was that she was overweight. She was following a food regimen that was providing her with too much fat. But it was the diet on which she had been brought up. Her parents ate the same foods she was eating. She was raised on those foods. Her parents had developed problems, too. This child was the recipient of her mother and father's neglect in taking care of their own bodies due to a lack of knowledge. Her body's inherent weaknesses were just added to an already bad condition. It is this kind of situation in which I would like to call a time out and conduct a class on proper nutrition. It is at this point that we have to think about eating properly. The bowel responds to good food within twelve to fifteen hours. Digestion in the small intestine and elimination in the large colon—the body must carry out these functions properly in order for us to have a healthy life. We can't let problems go until tomorrow. Tomorrow may be too late because by then we may be on our way to developing a toxic settlement in the body.

So, to take care of this overweight lady, I first had to look at the condition she was in today and the nutrition that could be used to make changes in that condition. Second, I had to look at the inherent weaknesses that were passed on to her from her mother and father.

One thing that we have to realize is that the human body molds to its environment. The body molds to a salad; it molds to coffee and donuts; it molds to the air we breathe; it molds to the water we drink. We must use our intelligence, our knowledge, and our wisdom to overcome the negative things in our environment and undertake a healthier way of life.

We have to make changes. We have to move away from our thinking of last year or twenty years ago. It may be time now to cut the umbilical cord and stop doing as Mother and Father did. We must realize that sometimes our lifestyle is quite self-destructive. This is because of the foolishness so common in human beings, because of the neglect and the ignorance to which we are prone.

If there is one way that is better than others, it's the way of nature. The best is not always what science tells us to do, or what a doctor tells us to do. Better than looking toward science or doctors is turning to nature for a new and better understanding.

Chapter 1

Raising Our Bowel Consciousness

As out of dirty mud-beds, gorgeous lilies grow—
so out of bent-old-age, comes vibrant youth!
And youth from age, is not a greater miracle
than pure white lilies growing out of mud!

—"Two Miracles," Author unknown

In times past, knowledge of the bowel was more common, and people were taught how to care for the bowel. Somehow, bowel wisdom has been lost, and the bowel has become a subject about which no one wants to talk. By hiding the issue in the closet, people have created an "out-of-sight, out-of-mind" situation. Thus, many people follow the path of ignorance and improper living, treating the bowel indiscriminately and reaping a sad harvest in their later years. Knowing the methods of keeping the bowel healthy is the best way to avoid the grip of disease and sickness.

The bowel-wise person is the one who is armed with correct information, practices discrimination in eating, and walks the path of a healthier life. His or her days are marked by well-being, vitality, and optimism, all of which result from having a vital, toxin-free body due to the efficient, regular cleansing action of a well-cared-for bowel. If you desire the higher things in life, you must be aware of proper bowel management—what it is, how it works, and what is required. This awareness will help you discover many secrets of life, develop a positive attitude toward yourself, and become the master of your bodily functions.

9

The bowel responds well to the laws of right living described in this book. You must be aware of these laws and be diligent in following them. The rewards in well-being and freedom from disease are more than worth the effort.

Alvin Toffler, in his book *Future Shock*, aptly states that mankind's current and future survival require the ability to adopt new ideas and habits very quickly—in fact, much more quickly than has ever been managed in the past. Is mankind up to it?

I believe that the number-one source of the misery and decay we are witnessing in our society today is autointoxication—self-poisoning caused by microorganisms, metabolic waste, and other toxins in the body. Through autointoxication, the human body becomes the unwitting host of uncleanliness with its entourage of imbalance, derangements, perversions, sickness, and disease. Autointoxication becomes a powerful master over the body, robbing the inhabitant of clear thinking, discrimination, sound judgment, vitality, health, and happiness. The ultimate rewards of autointoxication are disillusionment, bitterness, disappointment, chaos, and failure. Are you willing to make changes and do something about it? Overcoming the effects of autointoxication can be a long and difficult task, one often tragically postponed. However, it is preferable to correct autointoxication at the beginning rather than to struggle with its consequences later in life. I believe in educating, not medicating. A lack of education early on will necessitate medication as time passes.

Through education, we learn that healing takes place in accordance with one of the most important laws I have followed in my sanitarium work. This is Hering's Law of Cure, which was formulated by the nineteenth-century European homeopathic physician Constantine Hering. As Dr. Hering worked with the natural principles of healing, he came to see a great truth. He expressed it this way: "All cure starts from within out, from the head down, and in the reverse order as the symptoms appeared." Hering's Law is a most reliable guide to the natural healing process and worthy of reiteration at appropriate points in this book.

If we begin our search for a cure by using our heads, we come to understand that the bowel is one of the first things that has to be managed in our body-maintenance program. No one has ever had a home, office, or similar facility in which the elimination of wastes was not a consideration. Wastes, whether they be organic or otherwise, are a natural result of the process of living.

Years ago, it was found that many of mankind's diseases came from the poor handling of wastes or lack of proper sanitation. People would let urine, kitchen wastes, and bowel eliminations just run in the street gutters. This situation played a major role in spreading the many diseases and plagues that were once prevalent in Europe and various places throughout the world. Over the centuries, sanitation has been improved in many ways. In the cities, underground sewers take away the potentially harmful wastes of the population. In rural areas, septic systems have replaced the old outhouses, an improvement in convenience as well as sanitation. Cleansing agents and bactericides are used routinely to disinfect office buildings and homes. In these respects, we've come a long way.

We find, however, that to take care of bodily waste elimination, we must start within. We must stop allowing unsanitary conditions and their effects to develop in our bodies through unhealthy food choices and thoughtless lifestyles. We have a sanitation department in the body. We have a cesspool or a sewer, so to speak, and we must keep it clean. We must learn to take proper care of our inner environment so that we can avoid disease and encourage health.

It is ironic that in spite of our modern external sanitation, we give precious little thought to taking care of our personal internal sanitation. We know that Grandma always took care of the bowel. She would use a mixture of sulfur and molasses, one of the old remedies. She would also use enemas to clear a congested bowel. In days past, people were more familiar with bowel problems and the methods of remedying them. We've gotten away from doing these things today, and many people are suffering unnecessary sickness and disease because of it.

EDUCATING INSTEAD OF MEDICATING

If we lived correctly, we would have no need to concern ourselves with the bowel. However, most of us do not live correctly. We don't eat the right foods, we don't get the right exercise, and we don't get enough fresh air and sunshine. There are so many things we don't do correctly, we can't expect the bowel to function correctly.

When we look at the statistics on disease today and what doctors are doing about the situation, we see that much attention is directed at treating problems and troubles that are the result of bad lifestyle habits. Bad habits are the result of a lack of education. People just do what everyone else does, and few there are who have any other knowledge.

All that is modern is not necessarily good. Bad habits are too often picked up from modern civilization. When I say "modern civilization," I'm talking about progress. We all like to think of ourselves as progressive people, but it is obvious that a lot of the things we've progressed to are not always so good for our health. Air pollution is contributing to increased lung problems. The purity of our drinking water is being compromised by chemicals leaching from the soil or introduced deliberately to kill harmful bacteria. Even the toilet is a modern convenience that is not as good as it should be. (See "Complications of the Modern Toilet" on page 150.) We can do better.

Doctors are not teaching people to live correctly, and they must begin to make changes. After all, the very title "Doctor" is derived from the Latin *docere*, which means "to teach." I believe that every doctor should spend half of his or her time teaching patients how to promote good health. Doctors need to take the responsibility for educating patients because knowledge is an essential part of the healing process. When you are hospitalized for a health condition that was created by your lifestyle and dietary habits, as most conditions are, it isn't enough to be patched up and sent home to make the same mistakes over again. People in hospitals should never be discharged until they are given a full day of education in the management of their kitchens at home, nutrition for their families, and prevention of the recurrence of the trouble that brought them there. Otherwise, they are candidates for return visits.

There are too many people with a coffee-and-doughnut lifestyle who go to the doctor, get a treatment, and then go right back to their caffeine-and-sugar habit. They will be back. You can count on it. The doctor is counting on it, too. He will be counting all the way to the bank! You may think I'm being a little harsh, but every doctor admits that one operation leads to another. Do you know why? Because nothing is done to deal with the problems that lead to first operation.

Consider the following paraphrase of an article I read in a major daily newspaper: Of the 22,000 people diagnosed yearly as having colon cancer (with cancer also in the lymph nodes), most are treated surgically. Medical experts claim that over half of these patients would benefit from receiving an anticancer medication called 5-fluorouracil, plus a second medication called levamisole, after surgery. You see, the modern answer to these health problems is the utilization of medications.

The American Cancer Society has expressed the idea that it may take twenty years or more for some cancers to develop. With due appreciation of the progress being made with cancer medications and surgical techniques, I'd like to ask where the doctor was twenty years ago when the cancer was starting? Why is our healthcare system placing so much emphasis on treatment and so little on prevention? If we took a survey and asked a million people whether they would prefer to receive treatment for cancer or never get the disease in the first place, what do you think they would say? We need to learn how to take better care of ourselves from the preventive standpoint.

What do government health departments do? Mainly, they watch for and keep records about disease. Their focus is disease. They would more correctly be referred to as "disease departments." When an epidemic comes along, they try to figure out where it began, how it is spreading, and what the appropriate treatments are. With the possible exception of recommending inoculations, they do little to prevent epidemics.

We give money to organizations and institutions that are concerned with a particular disease condition, but do these groups spend any time trying to find out how to prevent the disease? I see that one organization was given a sizable grant to study diet and nutrition and their effects on cancer. The organization was going to start its research by studying alcohol's effects on already-established cancers. I believe it is reasonable to ask why the group chose not to conduct research to find out how to help prevent cancer. It goes without saying that the finding will be that alcohol has a detrimental effect. But this is still not going to tell us much about preventing cancer.

If we give money just to cure-oriented research, we will never understand how powerfully effective prevention can be. We must turn around. We must develop a new perspective in the way we look at health. We must make a concentrated effort to examine health strategies from the standpoint of prevention.

It is better to educate than medicate. I repeat this often because it is a fact that the more health education we have, the less medication we will need. We need to know how to become healthy and stay healthy. There are many different kinds of people, and we need to reach all of them at their own levels of understanding. Some people will pay anything to get well after they have become sick. However, we find that no matter how much money we may have, we cannot buy health. It's not for sale by anyone at any price. The truth is that you have to earn health. You must work for it. But too often, today's healthcare approach leaves the patient devoid of knowledge, with no change of consciousness, understanding, or behavior. Unless you elevate your mental attitude, your consciousness, you cannot reach a higher plane of health. This is accomplished through education. You can begin your education by learning about the body's channels for the elimination of waste.

THE FIVE MAIN ELIMINATION ORGANS

This book deals primarily with what I call the king of all the elimination organs, the bowel. It would be neglectful, however, if we did not give some consideration to the other four. It has been reaffirmed that the body functions as a whole, which requires that each component part do its work. If any of the five main elimination organs functions below par, it places an extra load upon the others in the body's effort to get rid of its metabolic waste material.

In addition to the bowel, there is the skin, the largest elimination organ. Taking care of the skin and ensuring that it functions well helps to relieve the other elimination organs. Skin brushing (see page 118) is suggested as a way of removing dead skin cells and the waste material excreted through perspiring.

Next are the kidneys, which are so important to our internal cleanliness that we have been provided with them in duplicate. We have a 100-percent-reserve in the ability to filter our blood of toxic waste and excess water. A person can lose the complete function of one kidney and still live because the other one, if it is functioning well, has the ability to carry the load alone. Perhaps one kidney can do the job because the skin acts as a supplemental filter, removing wastes from the blood. The finest way to aid the kidneys is to drink plenty of clean water. Drinking watermelon juice will also aid the kidneys in their elimination job.

Another main channel of elimination is the lymphatic system. The lymph has the job of picking up intracellular waste and dumping it into the bloodstream, where it is then processed by the liver and filtered by the kidneys. White blood cells in the lymph also destroy harmful bacteria as part of their function in the body's immune system. Unlike blood, lymph has no pump to force it through its vessels, which extend to every corner of the body. Lymph circulation depends upon movement of the extremities and muscle action. That's why most of our lymph nodes are concentrated in the places of greatest movement in the body. They are found where the arms and legs meet the torso and in the neck at the spot where nearly constant movement occurs. Is it any wonder, then, that exercise is of the greatest benefit to the lymph?

Last, but not least, are the lungs and bronchioles, considered together as part of the respiratory system. Some of the toxic waste material generated in the body is passed out of the system as a gas through the lungs. Carbon dioxide is exchanged for oxygen during the process of breathing. Once again, exercise comes into play as a natural way of increasing elimination. The finest exercise for the lungs is sniff breathing (see below). Developed by the late Robert Gaines and described in his book *Vitalic Breathing*, sniff breathing has been taught to members of the New York City Police Department to enhance their stamina by increasing their lung capacity. Improved exchange of gasses results in better oxygenation of the blood and better removal of toxic wastes.

During my many years of sanitarium work, I have found that taking care of the five main elimination systems is the most important thing we can do to gain and maintain health. Nothing is more important than making sure these five systems are working optimally. Neither all the medicines nor all the therapies in the world will help much or provide any lasting relief if these systems are not functioning well. The greatest, and the most abused and neglected, of all of these systems is the bowel.

Sniff Breathing

Sniff breathing is an exercise developed by Robert Gaines, author of the book *Vitalic Breathing*, which is no longer in print. Mr. Gaines taught the following exercise to members of the New York City Police Department to help increase their vital lung capacity:

1. Walk three steps while sniffing only through the nose using short, rapid inhalations. Sniff deeper with each step.

2. On the fourth step, exhale rapidly and completely.

3. For the next three steps, hold your breath.

4. Exhale completely on the eighth step.

5. Repeat steps 1 through 4.

Do this exercise three times daily, for five minutes at a time, for one month. Then increase it to four times daily, for eight minutes at a time.

OPERATING ON THE PROBLEM INSTEAD OF THE PERSON

I ask my patients what operations they've had and, almost invariably, the first was a tonsillectomy. The tonsils, a specialized lymphoid tissue, function to eliminate the matter generated during the body's fight against infection. They aid in the removal of wastes that occur in the body due to infection. An inflammation or enlargement of the tonsils indicates that the body is trying to throw off an overload of waste material. The tonsils excrete this material into the pharynx area, where it is swallowed and then passed out with the regular bowel movement. Removing the tonsils compromises the elimination system in the body because it forces other excretory pathways to do the job the tonsils once did.

Until fairly recently, it was the medical fashion to remove the tonsils routinely because they were believed to be a source of infection. Physicians believed that if the tonsils had a tendency to become inflamed, removing them would prevent them from becoming problematic. Due to the ignorance of the day, it was not realized that cutting out inflamed and enlarged tonsils is like ripping out a ringing fire alarm instead of attending to the fire. Tonsillitis is a sure warning that the body is overwhelmed by the need to eliminate waste materials. Today, some women with a family history of breast cancer are using the same logic. They're having their healthy breasts, which also contain a lot of lymph tissue, removed. Have we just traded one ignorance for another?

The next-most-common operation is the appendectomy. Considered a vestigial organ by medical authorities, the little wormlike appendix, like the tonsils, is another example of lymphoid tissue. It, too, can become inflamed if it is overburdened and toxic, as is common when the colon is dysfunctional and toxic, because the appendix is attached to the colon.

Toxic-colon problems, including appendicitis, occur when we fail to keep our bodies clean—that is, clean on the inside. The problem is that most people don't know how to keep clean on the inside. We are bombarded with advertisements for all types of products that clean the outside of the body, but no one tells us how to clean the inside. We do not need to pay more attention to external cleanliness; we need to pay more attention to internal cleanliness, to the body's internal environment. We can't put clean food into a dirty body and expect good results. We're going to get only partial, perhaps even negligible, results. We must go beyond clean food. True cleanliness begins on the inside. It begins with a clean thought, a higher consciousness. Next, we move to the physical plane, remembering that a person will

become on the outside what he thinks on the inside. We must cultivate a clean mind and, with it, clean body tissues. Cleanliness of mind
is a spiritual effort; the physical job begins with bowel care.

We have been educated to believe that if the bowel doesn't function correctly, we can turn to laxatives. I read somewhere that more
laxatives are sold in the United States than any other medication with
the exception of aspirin. Over-the-counter cold remedies are also big
sellers, as are tranquilizers, but you will find laxatives in almost every
medicine chest. Someone in every family seems to be constipated,
seems to have bowel problems. Before commercial laxatives were
available, other methods were used to stimulate the bowel.

In times past, when a child got sick, what did a mother do? Give
the child an enema, of course. Years ago more than today, people
knew the importance of bowel movements and their relationship to
good health. If a person had to resort to a laxative, he or she probably
used a mixture of sulfur and molasses. But we have found that laxatives are not a lasting or even a healthful solution to constipation. Our
knowledge of bowel care needs to go beyond the use of laxatives to
relieve constipation. We need to be sufficiently well-informed so that
we can avoid chronic bowel troubles. Unattended long enough, such
chronic problems may require surgical intervention. Let's operate on
the problem, not the person.

Education should give the mind a new or a greater sensitivity, an
appreciation that has been blocked by ignorance. A new sensitivity of
mind is needed in order to appreciate and care for the bowel. It is
especially worthy of note that the bowel has very few pain sensors,
very few nerves that carry sensory information to the brain to be
interpreted as pain. Abdominal surgeons will tell you that anesthesia
is needed in abdominal surgery mainly to enable a painless incision
of the abdominal wall. Once inside the abdominal cavity, surgeons
can handle the bowel without causing pain. The near absence of pain-
transmitting nerves makes it difficult for us to receive distress calls
from the bowel.

Contrast this to the heightened awareness of any problem on the
skin, an organ with a festival of nerves. For instance, the skin on our
lips is so imbued with touch and pain sensors that we can discern
something as fine as a single hair coming in contact with it. Consider
the skin in comparison to the bowel, and you will quickly realize
how vastly different one part of the body can be from another in the
ability to provide sensory input to the brain. By the time a bowel
problem is serious enough to cause pain, you can safely bet there is a
big problem.

Because of the low level of pain sensation in the bowel, the average person doesn't take care of the bowel until a problem becomes pronounced. The truth of this was especially brought home to me with the death of the popular movie actor John Wayne. You may remember that the first operation Mr. Wayne had was for lung cancer in 1964, after which he returned home. Later, he was back in the hospital, for an operation on cancer of the stomach, and was again sent home. More time passed and he had to return for yet a third operation, this one for cancer of the bowel. This was his final surgery, not long before his death in 1979. In my opinion, his bowel should have been checked carefully at the earliest sign of cancer in his lungs.

Since my main point in this book is that the condition of the bowel is related to conditions in all the other parts of the body, we should look to the bowel first, not last. I'm as sure as I can be from my experience with so many others that there was bowel trouble in John Wayne's case a long time before there was any problem in his stomach or lungs. If his bowel had been taken care of earlier, problems might not have occurred elsewhere. The only way to avoid problems is to educate ourselves to care for the bowel properly because the bowel is often disastrously tardy in "speaking for itself." If we learn to care for the bowel, we can avoid the many conditions associated with a toxic colon.

HOW A TOXIC COLON AFFECTS THE BODY

I believe that when the bowel is underactive, toxic wastes are more likely to be absorbed through the bowel wall and into the bloodstream. The blood then circulates these toxins to every part of the body and deposits some of them in tissues. The greatest amounts of toxins are retained in the constitutionally weakest tissues. If any other elimination system is underactive, more wastes are retained in the body. As toxins accumulate in the tissues, alterations in cellular function take place, especially in the tissues in which toxins have settled. In addition, digestion may become poor, with the partially digested material adding to the problem because the body cannot make tissue out of half-digested nutrients. When a person reaches the degenerative-disease stage, it is a sign that toxic settlements have taken over a specific part or parts of the body. This is the time to consider detoxification, the cleansing of the body tissues.

The body can be overwhelmed by toxic accumulations as a consequence of fatigue, poor circulation, or improper diet. When we undertake to detoxify the body, we must take care of those things in particular to avoid simply spinning our wheels. I want to emphasize that an underactive body burdened with toxic wastes does not have the capability to throw off toxins. As a body becomes increasingly toxic, proper oxygenation cannot take place in the tissues. Without oxygen, the body loses energy, and the tired body continues its downward spiral. A tired body has a reduced ability to throw off toxins, which is why toxic, sick people are always tired people.

WORKING TOWARD A HEALTHY BOWEL

Of all the processes essential to good health, elimination is certainly one of the most important. And when we consider the systems of the body, it is apparent that the gastrointestinal system is very important. I must admit that I didn't realize the importance of good bowel care until years of experience in clinical nutrition proved to me, beyond the shadow of a doubt, that the condition of the bowel tissue is often the key to the state of health or disease of the person.

I am convinced that our problems begin more often in the bowel than in any other part of the body. The body depends on a clean bowel. Remember, the cleanliness of any tissue in the body depends upon the condition of the bowel. When we arrive at the point where we realize these simple facts, we have come a long way toward raising our bowel consciousness.

Perhaps because of the bowel's paramount importance among the elimination organs, some health professionals have already become bowel-minded. Although we have discovered that it is much better to be whole-body-minded, we need to start our tissue detoxification beginning with the bowel. To accomplish this, we need to make sure that the bowel has sufficient water, good nerve tone, good muscle tone, adequate circulation, and the correct biochemical nutrients in the proper amounts. But we cannot build or maintain a good bowel if it is toxic-laden and dirty. Cleansing must come first.

Tissue laced with internal (metabolic) toxins or external toxins (from polluted air or water, or tobacco smoke) can't assimilate nutrients well or eliminate its own wastes efficiently. If injured, toxin-laced tissues heal extremely slowly until they are cleansed of those toxins. The bowel is the source of most internal toxic material, which makes its way into the blood and lymph through the bowel wall and is then carried to and deposited in the tissues. A cleaner bowel leads to cleaner blood, which leads to cleaner tissues, which then rebuild more easily.

Rebuilding is not an easy task and should not be thought of as a "quick fix" solution. I don't believe anyone can do a good job in less than a year's time. We must allow time for the proper foods to replenish the body's reserves between cleansings. Most people, if they think about it, know that good and lasting results take time. This is something to think about in this age of fast cars, fast food, and the fast buck.

According to statistics compiled by the Registrar General of England, no group has contributed more to the death rate from intestinal diseases than doctors. These statistics show that the death rate of doctors is higher than those of both agricultural workers and the English population in general. Is there any way that these troubles can be avoided? Yes, there is. Medical science touts early detection, but the real job is one of prevention. When we are young, we need to learn how to care for the bowel, and that includes making changes in the ways we live and eat.

The Registrar General's statistics ought to be telling us something. Are we going to wait, persisting in our business-as-usual frame of mind and hope that "early" detection will save us if we become a statistic? Are we trusting that the doctors will save us when it is obvious that they don't do a very good job of saving themselves? It is time that we take it upon ourselves to learn what we can do to help ourselves.

A BRIEF LESSON ON THE ANATOMY AND PHYSIOLOGY OF THE BOWEL

Although proper bowel management does not require us to become bowel experts, raising our bowel consciousness does necessitate our understanding the basic essentials of bowel anatomy (structure) and physiology (function).

The Small Intestine

When food leaves the stomach during the digestive process, it enters the long coiled tube known as the small intestine. By the time it reaches the small intestine, it has been reduced by the action of chewing and by digestive juices into a semiliquid known as chyme (pronounced *kime*, rhyming with "lime"). With the help of hormonal secretions, the small intestine digests and assimilates nutrients through its wall. The small intestine is the site of approximately 90 percent of the absorption of nutrients into the bloodstream.

Carbohydrates are digested beginning in the mouth, where they are broken down during chewing by enzymes in the saliva. Proteins are broken down into amino acids in the stomach, with further reduction taking place in the small intestine. All food elements are broken down to a size at which they can be properly absorbed. Of course, some elements, such as fiber, cannot be broken down or absorbed at all. These nonabsorbable elements, as we will see in Chapter 2, still have an important function, however.

When the chyme has been thoroughly mixed and broken down in the stomach, the pyloric sphincter opens and allows it to enter the duodenum, the uppermost section of the small intestine. Here, it is again thoroughly mixed and further broken down to prepare it for absorption by the intestinal villi. Specifically, longitudinal and circular muscles in the intestinal walls perform three different types of movements to process the chyme. The first type of movement is rhythmic segmentation, in which numerous adjacent circular muscles contract to segment the food as it passes. These muscles contract in sets, with one set of muscles contracting while another relaxes. As this muscular action is repeated, multiple squeezing actions take place twelve to sixteen times a minute. As a result of these movements, the chyme is thoroughly mixed with the digestive juices. The second type of movement is a wavelike contraction that travels forward and then in reverse over the length of a few centimeters of the intestine. This movement sloshes the chyme back and forth for intensive mixing. The third type of movement is known as peristalsis. Peristalsis is a large wavelike contraction of the intestine caused by the rhythmic flexing of muscles. Unlike the sloshing actions that facilitate mixing, peristalsis helps to propel the chyme through the small intestine.

These normal muscular activities of the intestine are not usually felt, although toxin-producing bacteria may cause violent and painful spasms. Awareness of the normal muscular actions of the digestive process would be uncomfortable and annoying. However, it is the lack of sensory input to the brain from the intestinal area that often lulls us into assuming that all is well with the bowel when, in fact, it may not be.

When the chyme first enters the duodenum from the stomach, it is highly acidic. It contains a concentration of hydrochloric acid and enzymes that breaks down the larger protein molecules to facilitate further digestion and absorption. The secretions of the small intestine contain bicarbonate, an alkaline substance, which neutralizes the stomach acid. In the pancreatic duct, which joins the common bile duct, the chyme is also mixed with pancreatic juice before it empties into the duodenum. Pancreatic juice contains several digestive enzymes and helps to further break down proteins, carbohydrates, and fats. Within the small intestine, bile salts, produced in the liver and then concentrated and stored in the gallbladder, act like a detergent to emulsify the fats, thus facilitating their absorption.

About 80 percent of the fluid in the body is made up of sodium-rich lymph and fluids other than red blood. Some of these fluids carry nutrients and toxic wastes just as the blood does. Their cleanliness depends upon the cleanliness of the bowel. The life of all the cells in the body depends upon the quality and cleanliness of the fluid that bathes them.

The small intestine is so constructed that nutrient absorption is highly efficient. A large inner surface area is provided by accordion-like folds in the intestinal wall. The average adult has a small-intestine area of approximately two hundred square feet. Lining the intestinal wall are fingerlike projections called villi, which extend into the interior of the intestine from all directions. The villi contain blood capillaries and lymph capillaries. The small molecular particles of the broken-down food are able to pass into the villi, where they are taken up by the tiny blood capillaries. They are transported to the hepatic portal vein and then to the liver, where they are reduced even further. From the liver, the digested nutrients are delivered to other cells in the body to support the life-giving cellular activities.

Fat particles, however, do not always enter the bloodstream this way. Unlike protein and carbohydrate particles, they can also be absorbed in a second way. The way in which they are absorbed depends upon whether they are composed more of long chemical chains or short chemical chains. Both kinds of fat are taken up from the intestine through the villi, but longer-chain fatty acids are broken down into triglycerides, which are then absorbed, in the form of minute droplets known as chylomicrons, from the villi into the lymphatic system. The chylomicrons are carried by the lymph system to the thoracic duct, which is where they enter the bloodstream through a large vein in the neck called the superior vena cava. The shorter-chain fatty acids, which make up about 10 to 20 percent of all fats, are absorbed directly into the portal vein, bypassing the lymph system. Both longer- and shorter-chain fatty acids end their journey by passing through the liver, where they are desaturated (metabolically rearranged) in preparation for conversion to energy.

In the final section of the small intestine, called the ileum, the chyme passes nodules of lymphoid tissue known as Peyer's patches. Named for their discoverer, the eighteenth-century Swiss anatomist Johann Conrad Peyer, these lymphoid tissues contain scavenger cells called lymphocytes that attack and destroy any unfavorable bacteria that may have found their way into the small intestine. The small intestine averages twenty to twenty-two feet in length and is from one-and-one-quarter to one-and-one-half inches in diameter. After the ileum, which is located in the lower right section of the abdomen, comes the large intestine.

The Large Intestine

Within eight to ten hours of being eaten, food is finished passing through the small intestine. It then enters the large intestine for the final digestive processes and elimination.

In contrast to the small intestine, in which there is very little bacterial action when healthy, the large intestine literally swarms with billions of microscopic organisms. Bacterial action in the large intestine plays a major role in nutrition and digestion. Friendly bacteria synthesize valuable nutrients such as vitamin K and some of the B vitamins by digesting portions of the bowel contents. This aspect of function is not completely understood and is being studied further. Any remaining proteins are broken down by the bacteria into simpler substances. There are numerous byproducts of this bacterial activity, such as indole, skatole, hydrogen sulfide, fatty acids, methane gas, and carbon dioxide. Some of these substances are very toxic and odorous, hence the smell that accompanies feces.

The large intestine is divided into sections called the cecum, ascending colon, transverse colon, descending colon, sigmoid colon,

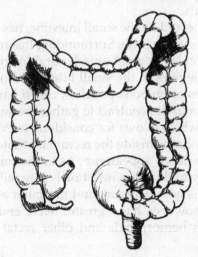

Figure 1.1. A healthy, normally functioning large intestine.

and rectum. A healthy, normally functioning large intestine is depicted in Figure 1.1. The cecum is a blind pouch located in the lower right abdomen. From the cecum, the large intestine rises up as the ascending colon until it reaches the first turn toward the left. Because of its proximity to the liver, this turning point is called the hepatic flexure. From here, the large intestine travels across the abdomen beneath the stomach until it reaches the second turn, called the splenic flexure, so named because this downward turn is near the base of the spleen. This section of the large intestine, the transverse colon, is the only organ that traverses the body from right to left. In a normal large intestine, the transverse colon also angles upward slightly as it crosses the body to the splenic flexure.

From the splenic flexure, the large intestine angles down as the descending colon until it reaches the sigmoid colon, which is just above the rectum. The sigmoid colon is the holding place for feces waiting to be eliminated. The rectum is the last segment of the large intestine as it continues from the sigmoid, making an S-like bend into the anus. The anal sphincter muscle serves to close off the large intestine, relaxing at will to allow feces to pass out as bowel evacuation becomes necessary. Altogether, the large intestine is approximately five feet long and two-and-one-half inches in diameter.

Also found in the large intestine is the ileocecal valve. Located in the cecum, where the cecum meets the small intestine, the ileocecal valve is a sphincter muscle that controls the flow of food wastes from the small intestine into the large intestine. Also situated here is the wormlike sac called the appendix. The appendix is about three inches long and, in many people, becomes inflamed—a condition that is known as appendicitis.

The large intestine, unlike the small intestine, has a mucous lining that is smooth and devoid of villi. Surrounding this mucous layer is a coat consisting of circular internal muscles and longitudinal external muscles similar to the ones in the small intestine. The large intestine is shaped like a series of bulbous pouches, called haustra. The circular and longitudinal muscles contract to gather the large intestine into accordionlike folds, which allows for considerable expansion.

The mucous membrane inside the rectum is striated in lengthwise segments, giving it a fluted appearance. As in the small intestine, the sensory-nerve supply to the large intestine is generally sparse. Therefore, pain or feeling is nearly absent, and muscular activity is largely unfelt. The rectum, however, has a greater nerve endowment, so the pain associated with hemorrhoids and other rectal disturbances is more readily felt.

Through the ileocecal valve, chyme is passed into the cecum from the small intestine. At this stage, the chyme consists of undigested and indigestible food substances; secretions from the liver, pancreas, and small intestine; and water. Most of the water in the chyme is absorbed in the cecum, reducing the chyme to a semisolid material called feces. To provide lubrication for the passage of the feces, numerous cells line the walls of the large intestine and secrete mucus.

With repeated peristaltic action, the feces are pushed toward the rectum and the anus, through which they are eliminated from the body. This movement is stimulated by the presence of food in the stomach. Peristalsis empties the cecum and makes it ready to receive new chyme from the small intestine.

When feces reach the rectum, they are about 65-percent water and 27-percent bacteria. The remaining 8 percent is made up of food residues, cellulose (fiber), indigestible materials, and dead cells discarded by the body. The time it takes for chyme to turn into feces in the cecum and travel to the rectum depends upon the amount of roughage and water in the food. Bulkier feces travel faster, as they provide substance upon which the bowel musculature can work. A soft, fiberless stool becomes very difficult for the bowel to move along. Furthermore, the longer it takes for feces to move, the more water is absorbed, making the feces compact and hard, and elimination becomes difficult.

Neglecting the urge to eliminate, as well as eating foods with little or no roughage, will lead to constipation. Laxatives taken to aid elimination often increase the amount of liquid retained in the feces or lubricate the feces to make their passage easier. Still other types of laxatives are compounded to be strong irritants. These laxatives stimulate the muscle walls to expel the irritating substances. It is very easy to become dependent upon any of the three basic types of laxative medications and thereby permanently destroy normal bowel function. Excessive use of laxatives can cause very watery feces or diarrhea, as can nervous stress, infection, or the presence of toxic substances in the bowel. Proper bowel management enhances the natural flow and rhythm of the digestive organs, providing regular, painless, and efficient functioning. When normal bowel function is compromised, the whole body is at risk.

Chapter 2

Intestinal Toxemia
and Autointoxication

Many obstacles interfere with the anatomical and physiological function of the idealized bowel described in the previous chapter. A deficient diet, an unhealthy lifestyle, and neglect of the natural urge to defecate are three of the most common obstacles. Improper bowel function leads to intestinal toxemia. When the intestinal tract is the recipient of an improper diet or when the colon is not evacuated in a timely fashion, the normal intestinal flora are replaced by more harmful bacteria, and intestinal toxemia is the inevitable consequence.

Autointoxication is the result of intestinal toxemia. Simply stated, autointoxication occurs when the body absorbs too much of its own toxic waste. Autointoxication is the outcome of an imbalanced diet and faulty bowel function, a combination that produces undesirable consequences in the body. It is the root cause of many of today's disorders and illnesses.

Creating the analogy of the large intestine as the body's waste-disposal unit or sewer system enables us to more clearly understand the ways in which the colon can malfunction. Imagine the result of a pump failure in a city's sewer system or of the pipes becoming plugged with some immovable material. It wouldn't be very long before a crisis developed and an ugly sanitation problem threatened the public health. From open sewers in the past sprang the devastating plagues and diseases that literally destroyed whole cities and populations. When the sewer backs up, we have an immediate health problem. Call the plumber!

In addition to the above scenario, there is the possibility that a power failure can bring a halt to the waste-elimination-and-treatment process. The works themselves are okay, but the energy that feeds all the machinery is shut off or cut back. We can compare this to what happens in our bodies when our food is nutritionally deficient and fails to give us adequate energy.

We experience all of the above conditions in our bowels today. Why? The full explanation would fill volumes. We can, however, distill the main causes for the sake of brevity and still get the message.

In modern civilization, the greatest numbers of bowel disturbances are found in the industrialized nations. We find that native peoples living close to the land and nature do not experience the problems and diseases associated with autointoxication. What is it that causes the bowel disturbances that are so prevalent in our culture? It's hard to point a finger at any one aspect in particular because there are many contributing factors. Some individuals react more intensely than others due to heredity, environmental factors, or personal living habits. In general, the overall major contributing factor is the straying away from a simple, natural lifestyle, wherein more of the preconditions for healthy living are found. The further we stray from natural processes and the more we depend on unnatural and artificial processes, the greater are the frequency and intensity of disease and illness.

The subject of intestinal toxicity is of wide-ranging clinical importance and should be emphasized. As will be made clear, intestinal toxemia is frequently found as either a basic cause of or a contributing factor to many clinical phenomena. Dr. Anthony Bassler, a professor of gastroenterology at Fordham University Medical College and New York Polyclinic Medical College and a consulting gastroenterologist at Christ's Polyclinic and People's Hospital in New York, conducted a twenty-five-year study of intestinal toxemia. In 1933, after having studied more than five thousand cases, he stated, "Every physician should realize that the intestinal toxemias are the most important primary and contributing causes of many disorders and diseases of the human body."

Intestinal toxemia is a process resulting from a certain type of diet or from intestinal obstruction. Various toxic chemicals are produced in the lumen (the space within an organ) by bacteria. These toxins are absorbed into the bloodstream in one of two ways. In one way, a toxin escapes the detoxifying action of the liver because of a pathological, functional insufficiency of the liver. In this case, the liver cannot act upon all of the toxins present. In the second way, a toxin escapes due to a physiological characteristic of the liver. Here, the liver normally does not act upon this particular toxin. The toxins then enter the general circulation and exert their deleterious effects before being excreted by the kidneys. The toxicity produces a pathological change in the tissues or aggravates a previously existing condition.

As part of his research on the subject of intestinal toxemia, Alan Immerman, D.C., a chiropractor with experience in natural therapeutics and detoxification, researched the medical literature from the years 1879 to 1978. He found that almost no clinically oriented articles about intestinal toxemia were written in the English language after the late 1950s. In fact, few papers that directly address this subject have been published since 1940. The probable reason for the neglect of the topic is the introduction of antibiotics into general use in the 1950s.

Back in 1928, the discovery of penicillin was hailed as the crowning achievement of modern medicine. For the first time in history, the bacterial infections responsible for thousands of deaths could be finally and totally conquered, it was touted. Penicillin and the antibiotics that followed it were used freely and with abandon. The age-old problems of gonorrhea and syphilis, exacerbated by World Wars I and II, were thought to have been beaten. No longer was it found necessary to modify the behavior of soldiers on shore leave when a simple shot in the buttocks was all that was needed to assure their safety. No one imagined that strains of bacteria resistant to the new "wonder drugs" would develop. Nor was it even remotely suspected that uncontrolled use of these miracle medications would result in compromising of the immune system. The doctors and the populace of the time were so confident in the future of the new medications that most abandoned, and in time forgot, the time-honored principles of cleanliness, conduct, and conservative care that their medical forbears had fought so hard to institute.

The new medications became the be-all and end-all of the modern, post–World War II era. Pharmaceutical companies expanded rapidly in the years following the war, and the burgeoning medico-pharmaceutical complex thought it was on its way to conquering disease through modern chemistry. The feeling was that chemistry had the world by the tail. With the power of the public's new affection backing them, the products spawned by the research in the chemical laboratories pushed aside the principles of proper diet and good bowel hygiene, principles that had once been considered good medicine. Little did anyone suspect that, in time, Mother Nature would exact her revenge for such foolhardiness in the face of her immutable laws. It is now time to turn our attention back to Mother Nature and the basics.

OBSTRUCTIVE INTESTINAL TOXEMIA

I mentioned previously that intestinal toxemia is a process resulting from improper diet or obstructive conditions in the bowel. To gain a better understanding of intestinal toxemia in general, we should first consider the more extreme cases of intestinal obstruction. Obstruction in the intestine is the cause of toxemia only in a very small percentage of cases. However, it is far more likely to be rapidly fatal than toxemia resulting from diet-related intestinal stasis. Studying the obstructive type may, however, give us insights into extreme situations.

Obstruction can be surgically created in laboratory animals by the formation of a closed intestinal loop. The loop is washed to exclude the secretions of the stomach, liver, and pancreas, along with the products of food digestion. The loop is then surgically closed. The result has been the same in all experiments. The bacteria multiply greatly, and the proteolytic bacteria (the bacteria involved in protein breakdown) overgrow all the others, producing toxic chemicals in the process. These toxins are absorbed, and the animals become sick and rapidly succumb to toxic shock, which is characterized by low blood pressure, kidney failure, and liver malfunction. The toxins produced include histamine, which is normally present in all cells but becomes highly concentrated in the presence of an intestinal obstruction, and protein-decomposition products, which vary in toxicity.

During experiments, the toxins produced in the closed intestinal loop have been removed and injected into healthy animals. This action has resulted in a more intense but similar condition to what developed in the animals with the surgically closed loops. When the toxins were injected into the portal vein, they were transported directly to the liver. The finding was that the liver plays no essential role in detoxifying these particular poisons. The poisons were produced by putrefactive bacteria that are normally present but that had multiplied greatly and overgrown all the other bacteria in the obstructed intestine. Given the condition of the experimental animals, it seems reasonable to suppose that toxins are produced and absorbed when intestinal stasis without total obstruction is coupled with high protein intake.

It is important to emphasize again that intestinal obstruction similar to that observed in animals with a surgically closed intestinal loop is rarely seen in people. Such complete obstruction is certainly not the basic cause of intestinal toxemia in most cases. However, insight into the process of intestinal toxemia can be gained by observations of the experimental extreme. This is the same logic used by researchers who

feed a suspected carcinogen to lab animals in quantities ten times greater than a human being could ever consume in the same time period.

Now let's consider some of the toxins resulting from intestinal
putrefaction associated with the action of bacteria as it breaks down
protein. Our focus is on protein because protein digestion produces
the most toxic metabolic products.

TOXIC CHEMICALS PRODUCED BY PROTEOLYTIC BACTERIA

To date, the exact nature of all the compounds formed by proteolytic
bacteria has not been completely identified. Unfortunately, along with
the development of instrumentation sophisticated enough to yield this
information, there has been a simultaneous loss of medical interest in
the subject of intestinal toxemia. This loss of interest is probably associated with the increased use of antibiotics to control bacterial overgrowth.

We do know that ammonia is one of the substances formed by the
action of proteolytic bacteria in the intestine. One of the functions of
the liver is to convert this ammonia into urea, which can then be
excreted by the kidneys. In liver dysfunction or disease, such as cir-
rhosis, or in blockage of circulation to the liver, abnormal levels of
ammonia may occur in the circulating blood. Corresponding but
lesser elevations of ammonia occur in the cerebrospinal fluid. An
increased concentration of ammonia in this fluid causes severe neurological symptoms such as mental disturbances, tremors, and an altered electroencephalograph (EEG) pattern. Increased concentrations
of ammonia in the blood induce hepatic (liver) coma and eventual
death. Coma and death are the result of various organs, including the
brain, becoming dysfunctional because increased toxic waste cannot
be detoxified and eliminated. It is even thought that excess levels of
ammonia may be involved in the malignant transformation of cells. A
low-protein diet is less taxing on the liver and, in liver disease, minimizes the symptoms of toxicity.

Modern medical opinion on ammonia is revealed in *Harrison's
Principles of Internal Medicine*, edited by Kurt J. Isselbacher, et al., in
which is stated:

> [B]oth hepatic coma and the chronic form of hepato-cere-
> bral disease are characterized by hyperammonemia, which
> is probably important in their pathogenesis. Ammonium is
> derived from the bacterial action on intestinal proteins and
> normally is converted to urea in the liver. Confusion,
> drowsiness, or other signs of impending hepatic coma,

should be treated by a prompt decrease in protein intake to levels of 20 to 30 grams daily or less.*

In plain English, this means that intestinal putrefaction associated with a high protein intake can place a high demand upon the liver. If the liver is not capable of detoxifying these protein metabolic wastes, serious health problems can result. Reducing protein intake is thus a part of a multidisciplinary approach to the treatment and management of liver dysfunction.

In addition to ammonia, clostridium perfringens enterotoxin is another highly toxic substance found among the putrefactive wastes of a compromised intestine. Clostridium is a type of bacteria, and the perfringens variety is known to cause dysentery in certain animals. An enterotoxin is a toxin specific to the cells of the intestinal lining.

Another substance, indole, is formed from tryptophan, again by the action of proteolytic bacteria. Tryptophan is one of the amino acids that compose protein. Experiments on animals as well as on humans have demonstrated that indole is toxic. Other tryptophan metabolites (substances that result from tryptophan metabolism) are also known to be toxic.

With normal liver function, most, if not all, toxic substances such as indole are detoxified or at least rendered less toxic by being chemically joined to other elements, a process known as conjugation. Conjugation is the primary way the liver renders toxic substances less harmful. In certain disease conditions, or when the body's major systems of elimination are overtaxed or have a significant degree of dysfunction, a high-protein, low-carbohydrate diet results in increased excretion of conjugated indole. Conjugated indole forms a new substance known as indican. Because the amount of indican excreted in the urine can be accurately determined by a laboratory test, its presence has been widely used as an indicator of intestinal putrefaction, but this determination alone is not adequate for making a positive diagnosis. When phenol (carbolic acid), a metabolite of the amino acid tyrosine, is tested for in addition to indican, the results more accurately point to intestinal putrefaction.

Phenol is so extremely poisonous that it is used as an antimicrobial agent. It is both a local corrosive and a systemic poison that can cause the destruction of the gastrointestinal lining as well as of kidney and liver cells. Phenol is absorbed into the blood from the intestine, and most of it is excreted in its free (unconjugated) form and, therefore, not detoxified. As with indole, the concentration of phenol in the urine increases with protein consumption.

Skatole is another toxic byproduct of bacterial action on tryptophan. It causes depression of the circulation and central nervous system, and is also found in increased concentrations in the intestine following a high protein intake. Skatole, when in excess in the circulating blood, imparts a foul odor to the breath. Skatole and indole are partially responsible for the characteristic odor of feces.

Hydrogen sulfide is another byproduct of protein decomposition. In comparable concentrations, it's as toxic as cyanide. It is not surprising that such a toxic gas is an irritant to the intestinal lining. Irritation from hydrogen sulfide brings about congestion and enables the intestinal contents, including intestinal toxins, to more easily penetrate the intestinal wall and be taken up by the blood. Poisoning by this gas will cause weakness, nausea, clammy skin, rapid pulse, and cyanosis (a blue tinge to the skin, especially the lips, caused by a lack of oxygen in the blood).

Aminoethyl mercaptan is formed from the bacterial decomposition of the amino acid cysteine. It has been observed to profoundly lower blood pressure. It is also very odorous. If you have experienced the telling odor of a natural gas leak in your home, you have smelled mercaptan. Natural-gas distributors add a small amount of mercaptan to their product so that people can detect the normally colorless and odorless natural gas. Mercaptan and other foul-smelling gases are created in the putrefactive bowel, and their uncontrolled escape, audible or not, can often result in social embarrassment.

Tyramine is a putrefactive product of tyrosine. It instigates the release of the hormone norepinephrine in the body. Norepinephrine narrows the blood vessels, thereby raising the blood pressure.

Scientists and researchers believe that putrefactive end products are irritants to the nerve endings in the intestinal wall. Because of this irritation, aberrant nerve impulses bombard the associated spinal-cord segments. When this happens, the organs or other areas of the body associated with these spinal segments are negatively affected. Therefore, not only the circulatory system but also the nervous system may be involved in passing along the adverse effects of bowel toxins to all the parts of the body.

Many other chemicals, too numerous to consider in detail, have been found to be formed in the intestine from bacterial putrefaction. Besides the known substances, many chemicals of unknown character may be produced. These chemicals may be toxic to various degrees.

Some may be completely detoxified by the liver, but others not at all. Other substances may be only partially rendered harmless. The highly complex subject of the chemistry of intestinal toxemia has been only partially researched and understood, whereas the situation from a clinical perspective, as we will see, is much clearer.

CLINICAL MANIFESTATIONS OF INTESTINAL TOXEMIA AND AUTOINTOXICATION

Sir W. Arbuthnot Lane, M.S., a fellow of the prestigious Royal College of Surgeons and a physician to England's royalty, was one of the most knowledgeable men to work with intestinal toxemia. (See "The Pioneering Work of Sir W. Arbuthnot Lane," below.) A surgeon with a penchant for the surgical treatment of intestinal toxemia, he observed

The Pioneering Work of Sir W. Arbuthnot Lane

Sir W. Arbuthnot Lane, the great English surgeon and physician to the English Crown who lived from 1856 to 1943, was one of the first to demonstrate that bowel troubles have a reflex effect upon specific organs in the body. He demonstrated that an irritation in the bowel can cause abnormal impulses to be sent via nerve pathways to a remote part of the body.

Dr. Lane spent many years specializing in bowel problems and was an expert at surgically removing sections of the bowel and stitching the healthy ends back together. He taught this work to other doctors and gained an international reputation for his efficiency. However, Dr. Lane began to notice a peculiar phenomenon. During the course of recovery from colonic surgery, some of his patients experienced remarkable cures of diseases that had no apparent connection to the surgery. For instance, a young boy who had had arthritis for many years had been using a wheelchair prior to his surgery. Six months later, this boy was entirely recovered from the arthritis. Another case involved a woman with goiter. When a specific section of her bowel was surgically removed, a definite remission of her goiter ensued within six months.

These and similar experiences impressed Dr. Lane greatly because he saw the relationship between the toxic bowel and the function of various organs in the body. After much thought about this relationship, he became very interested in changing the bowel through dietary methods and spent the last twenty-five years of his life teaching people how to care for the bowel through nutrition and not surgery.

Dr. Lane said, "All maladies are due to the lack of certain food principles, such as mineral salts or vitamins, or to the absence of the normal defenses of the body, such as the natural protective flora. When this occurs, toxic bacteria invade the lower alimentary canal, and the poisons thus generated pollute the bloodstream and gradually deteriorate and destroy every tissue, gland and organ of the body."

firsthand the pathological state of the intestines of many sick people. His therapy of choice, as might be suspected, was to remove the diseased section of the bowel. This was a successful method of providing temporary relief to the patient. As this book points out, however, unless corrections in bowel cleanliness, lifestyle, and diet are made, any attempts, surgical or otherwise, to cure the condition will be only temporary. Dysfunction will, in time, manifest itself again. As will be discussed later, other preventive and corrective measures are successful in giving permanent rather than temporary relief and are noninvasive—that is, they do not employ medications or surgery.

Dr. Lane defined chronic intestinal stasis as an "abnormal delay in the transmission of the intestinal contents through some portion or portions of the gastrointestinal tract, which delay may be accompanied by constipation or by a daily or even more frequent action of the bowels." He further stated that any such delay allows multiplication of undesirable organisms and the subsequent development of toxemia. This, he said, leads to "progressive degenerative changes in every tissue and a very definite and unmistakable series of symptoms." As has been mentioned, in cases of intestinal obstruction, bacteria multiply greatly, with the proteolytic bacteria overgrowing all the others. Is it not reasonable to consider that some features of chronic intestinal stasis are similar to but not as severe as those encountered in total obstruction?

Of great clinical importance is the fact that daily movement of the bowel alone cannot, contrary to popular belief, be considered evidence of proper bowel function. An experience of mine while I was attending the National College of Chiropractic in Chicago many years ago is illustrative of this fact. In the college anatomy laboratory, autopsies were performed on 300 bodies. According to the histories of these deceased persons, 285 had claimed they were not constipated and had normal bowel movements, and only 15 had admitted they were constipated. The autopsies, however, showed the opposite to be the case—only 15 were found not to have been constipated, while 285 were found to have been constipated. Some of the 285 persons had stated that they had as many as five or six bowel movements daily, yet the autopsies revealed that in some of them, the colon was twelve inches in diameter. The normal diameter of the colon is two to three inches. The bowel walls were encrusted with material (in one case, peanuts) that had been lodged there for a very long time. The average person does not know whether he or she is constipated. These observations beg for a more accurate and inclusive definition of constipation, a topic worthy of special consideration and one that will be discussed later. (See Chapter 3.)

Constipation is just one sign of an improperly functioning bowel. Donald V. Bodeen, D.C., Ph.D., my long-time student and a contributing researcher to this book, as well as my colleague and friend, has made a list of symptoms that are associated with intestinal toxemia and its resulting systemic autointoxication. It is interesting to note that his interest in bowel care is the result of his having himself suffered for many years from the effects of autointoxication. Because his doctors offered him only medications with no explanations of possible causes, Dr. Bodeen began his own search for an understanding of his ailments. This led to his compiling the following list of autointoxication symptoms:

❏ Headaches of various types   ❏ Drowsiness

❏ Back pain   ❏ Burning sensations in the
❏ Dementia   face, eyes, hands, or feet

❏ Depression   ❏ Tics (repetitious, sudden,
    involuntary movements)
❏ Forgetfulness

- ❏ Lack of ability to concentrate
- ❏ Stupor
- ❏ Indecision
- ❏ Bloating
- ❏ Fatigue
- ❏ Dermatological conditions
- ❏ Abdominal pain
- ❏ Dry eyes
- ❏ Tearing eyes
- ❏ Vision disturbances
- ❏ Sinus problems
- ❏ Abdominal cramps
- ❏ Heart arrhythmias (erratic heartbeats)
- ❏ Indigestion
- ❏ Nausea
- ❏ Hemorrhoidal pain
- ❏ Bad breath
- ❏ Body odor
- ❏ Foot odor
- ❏ Irritability
- ❏ Constipation
- ❏ Diarrhea
- ❏ Flatulence
- ❏ Coryza (common cold)
- ❏ Catarrh (inflammation of mucous membranes)
- ❏ Insomnia
- ❏ Fitful sleep
- ❏ Prolapse of abdominal organs
- ❏ Arthritis
- ❏ Photophobia (sensitivity to light)
- ❏ Pain behind the eyes
- ❏ Sensitivity to noise
- ❏ Melancholy
- ❏ Insanity
- ❏ Coma
- ❏ Delirium
- ❏ Cataracts
- ❏ Hypertension (high blood pressure)
- ❏ Hypotension (low blood pressure)
- ❏ Hardening of the arteries
- ❏ Appendicitis
- ❏ Inflammation or enlargement of the spleen
- ❏ Ovarian cysts
- ❏ Tumors
- ❏ Muscle atrophy
- ❏ Degeneration of organs
- ❏ Skin wrinkles
- ❏ Complexion alterations
- ❏ Boils
- ❏ Carbuncles
- ❏ Itching
- ❏ Acne
- ❏ Posture alterations
- ❏ Clammy skin
- ❏ Fallen arches
- ❏ Fibrocystic breasts

❑ Leg pains   ❑ Mastitis
❑ Malaise   ❑ Kidney disorders
❑ Twitching of muscles   ❑ Tonsil troubles
❑ Muscle inflammations   ❑ Bladder infections
❑ Degenerate, unclean thoughts   ❑ Bad dreams

This is to list but a few. Did you find your ailments on the list?

We can only begin to guess the number of people incarcerated in psychiatric facilities, prisons, and other institutions because of socially unacceptable behavior associated with mental dysfunction ultimately due to a filthy, toxic, and malfunctioning bowel. Our hospitals are jammed with people who have problems that are related to chronic toxic-bowel conditions, and neither the doctors nor patients suspect the true causes of the problems. Consider also the multitude who quietly suffer at home and at work on a daily basis, and those who are physically or psychologically addicted to the various medications and nostrums offered to alleviate their discomfort and otherwise mask their symptoms.

I am not claiming that every symptom in Dr. Bodeen's list arises from intestinal toxemia. However, the information should lead you to note that bowel toxemia is at the root of more problems than commonly imagined.

Generally, intestinal toxemia manifests as one or more of the following:

❑ Fatigue   ❑ Low-back pain
❑ Nervousness   ❑ Sciatica (inflammation of
❑ Gastrointestinal conditions   the sciatic nerve in the hip)
❑ Malabsorption of nutrients   ❑ Allergies
❑ Skin manifestations   ❑ Asthma
❑ Endocrine disturbances   ❑ Eye, ear, nose, and throat
❑ Neurocirculatory abnormalities   diseases
❑ Headaches   ❑ Cardiac irregularities
❑ Arthritis   ❑ Pathological changes in
                                      the breasts

All of these conditions have responded to therapy for intestinal toxemia.

You will note that I discuss only therapies aimed at relieving the toxic state of the intestine in general. To be more specific in each instance is beyond the scope of my intentions. The treatments mentioned are representative of those that have been used by many doctors, excluding the invasive treatments of surgery and medications. You will see that most of the incidents I cite are from the years prior to the discovery of antibiotics.

Allan Eustis, M.D., an instructor at Tulane University School of Medicine, reported in 1912 that 121 cases of bronchial asthma were relieved by eliminating the intestinal toxemia universally present. D. Rochester, M.D., of the University of Buffalo School of Medicine, stated in 1906 that after twenty-three years of observation, he concluded that toxemia of gastrointestinal-tract origin is the underlying cause of asthma. He said, "I believe the results of treatment justify my position."

Dr. Lane believed that arthritis could not develop in the absence of intestinal toxemia and said there is clinical and X-ray evidence of intestinal stasis in arthritis patients. Furthermore, he stated, "The symptoms disappear and the patients recover sometimes with startling rapidity when the condition of stasis has been effectually dealt with." Others confirm the connection between intestinal toxemia and arthritis. For example, Max Garten, D.C., N.D., in his book *"Civilized" Diseases and Their Circumvention*, claims that arthritis can be treated successfully with a fast immediately followed by a diet of raw foods and raw vegetable juices. "Severe arthritic involvements should be managed by alternating fasts or a vegetable juice regimen with a raw vegetarian food intake to the degree where at least 75% of the fare is raw or uncooked."

Not the least of the reasons for this regimen's success is that the high fiber content of raw vegetables decreases bowel transit time. Rapid transit means that substances are not in the intestine long enough to produce products of putrefaction. Furthermore, because vegetables are composed largely of complex carbohydrates, they do not produce nearly the amount of putrefactive wastes that foods high in protein do. Intestinal toxemia often tends to adversely influence the constitutionally weakest organ, system, or process in the body, which may include the heart.

Arthur C. Guyton, M.D., for many years a professor in and the chairman of the Department of Physiology and Biophysics at the University of Mississippi School of Medicine, states that "toxic conditions of the heart" can cause arrhythmias. Dr. Bodeen concurs. In the late 1980s, Dr. Bodeen reported on the particular case of a young female patient who had come to his office suffering from heart arrhythmias. Her symptoms were completely alleviated by cleansing her colon and modifying her diet to greatly improve a chronic toxic bowel. Prior to the diagnosis of chronic toxic bowel, the young woman had been unable to find the cause of her arrhythmias, although she had been hospitalized several times and had submitted to a number of the diagnostic studies used in orthodox medicine. It seems that no one had made the connection between a chronic toxic bowel and her episodic heart arrhythmias. The connection between these two conditions had been noted in 1916 by Dr. D.J. Barry, a professor of physiology at Queens College in Cork, England. Dr. Barry had stated, "There seems little doubt that substances having a deleterious action on the heart musculature and nerves are formed both in the small and large intestine, even under apparently normal circumstances."

The same principle applies to pregnancy. R.C. Brown, M.B., M.S., F.R.C.S., an obstetrical surgeon in England in 1930, linked intestinal toxemia and eclampsia, the latter commonly known as toxemia of pregnancy. Preeclampsia and eclampsia are conditions that develop as a complication of pregnancy. The conditions are characterized by a rise in blood pressure, the presence of albumin (protein substances) in the urine, and edema (swelling), which, if left untreated, can lead to coma and convulsive seizures. The cause is officially classified as unknown. But chronic toxemia's influence via the circulatory system and the nervous system can affect any part of the body.

Dr. Harold M. Peppard, in his very popular book *Sight Without Glasses*, says that eyestrain "is acute when the eyes are used, for example, during any severe toxic condition." He lists a number of acute toxic conditions, including the common cold. He points out that "people who 'catch up on their reading' while they are in bed with a cold are abusing their eyes as unmercifully as they would their bodies if they went on with their customary activities while running a temperature." If this is so, what effect does chronic bowel toxicity have on the eyes over a lengthy period?

C.A. Harter, M.D., a lecturer on the anatomy and pathology of the nervous system at New York Polyclinic, in 1892 linked intestinal putrefaction to epilepsy in 31 patients. He based his conclusion on the successful treatment of epilepsy using medications to control the bacterial activity of the intestine.

A toxic condition of the bowel is involved in many disorders of the nervous system. Drs. Satterlee and Eldridge, in a paper read to the annual session of the American Medical Association (AMA) in 1917, reported their experiences with 518 cases of "mental symptoms" including "mental sluggishness, dullness and stupidity; loss of concentration and/or memory; mental incoordination, irritability, lack of confidence, excessive and useless worry, exaggerated introspection, hypochondriasis and phobias, depression and melancholy, obsessions and delusions, hallucinations, suicidal tendencies, delirium and stupor." The doctors reported success in eliminating these symptoms by surgically relieving intestinal toxemia. During the discussion following the presentation of the paper, other physicians reported having had similar experiences. This is truly remarkable in light of today's commonly held beliefs.

Of considerable interest is a more recent paper, "Biochemical Aspects of Indole Metabolism in Normal and Schizophrenic Subjects," by Herbert Sprince. In this highly sophisticated paper, eleven independent laboratories are noted to have found at least five times more 6-hydroxyskatole in the urine of schizophrenics than in that of normal subjects. Such universal agreement, Sprince says, is highly significant, since this is an area where conflict, not agreement, is the rule. It is important to note that 6-hydroxyskatole arises primarily from skatole in the intestine, and that skatole arises from the action of putrefactive bacteria on tryptophan, as I previously mentioned.

Carl Von Noorden, M.D., a professor at the First Medical Clinic, Vienna, Austria, in 1913 found "pains especially frequent which correspond to the ordinary sciatic or intercostal neuralgia." Sciatic neuralgia is pain radiating down one or both legs, usually from the spinal nerves in the lower back. Intercostal neuralgia is pain in the chest, in the area between the ribs. Both these symptoms are common complaints. Dr. Noorden treated these conditions by relieving intestinal toxemia. Chiropractors see a lot of these conditions. Healthcare professionals would be well advised to review the facts on irritation to the nerves of the low-back area during a toxemic state of the intestine.

Various skin conditions have also been linked to intestinal toxemia. Dr. J.F. Burgess, M.M.B., a lecturer on dermatology at McGill University and associate dermatologist at Montreal General Hospital, reports the results of his study of 109 cases of eczema. He states that "on the basis of clinical observations and sensitivity tests against various amino acids and ptomaine bases, eczema is probably caused by intestinal toxemia." Dr. Bodeen and I both have had patients whose severe cases of psoriasis, an eczematous skin condition, cleared up following detoxification of the intestinal tract. Neither Dr. Bodeen nor I would go so far as to claim that intestinal toxemia is the *cause* of all psoriatic conditions, but would declare that there is a *strong association* between a toxic state of the bowel and many types of skin manifestations and eczematous conditions.

There are implications that intestinal toxemia may increase the

risk of cancer. Some physicians believe that the beginning of malignant disease in various organs comes within the wide range of conditions associated with intestinal stasis. Dr. Lane recorded his feeling of
being "exceedingly impressed by the sequence of cancer and intestinal stasis." In more recent years, the research of British surgeon Denis
P. Burkitt, M.D., has confirmed the lower incidence of several types of
cancer among eastern African natives eating a high-fiber diet, which
reduces bowel transit time. (See "Denis P. Burkitt, M.D." on page 52.)

Most medical doctors and health practitioners have long been
aware of the value of a high-fiber diet, which serves to increase intestinal motility. Late in the 1980s, the Kellogg Company, historically
associated with the late John Harvey Kellogg, M.D., and his famous
sanitarium, printed a statement about fiber's role in diet on the back
of its bran-cereal box: "A low-fat diet, rich in foods with fiber, may
reduce the risk of some forms of cancer." This was the first time
after many years that the U.S. Food and Drug Administration (FDA)
allowed a manufacturer to publicly make such a statement.

In its pursuit of the causes of and a cure for cancer, the medical
establishment has, in the past sixty years, turned away from the evidence and the convictions of respected physicians of an earlier time
that food habits and intestinal stasis are fundamental considerations
in understanding cancer. Recent research has focused on causes other
than diet, such as asbestos and cigarettes. The methods of cure have
been confined to surgery, radiation, and chemotherapy. The medical
establishment and its satellite institutions have created a powerful
paradigm for acceptable and unacceptable theories on the causes of
and cures for cancer. Any proposal that doesn't fit the paradigm is
thrown out. But, beginning in the 1970s, cracks have begun to appear
in the paradigm.

Research like a 1980 study at the University of California Medical
School in San Francisco revived the turn-of-the-century notion that
toxins in the bowel can have damaging effects on the body. The study
implied the possibility that bowel stasis is a cause of cancer. The find-
ings pointed to a link between a high-fat, low-fiber diet and an increased risk of breast cancer. The study of 1,481 non-nursing women
claimed that chronic constipation is linked to the abnormal cells found
in the fluid taken from the women's breasts. Previously, the same cells
had been found in women with breast cancer. These abnormal cells
were found five times more often in women who had fewer than three
bowel movements per week than in women who had more than one
bowel movement per day. Chronic constipation was recognized as
resulting more frequently with a diet high in protein, fats, and refined

carbohydrates than a diet high in fiber foods such as fruits, vegetables, and whole grains. In fact, constipation seemed to be conspicuously lacking among those who ate the latter diet.

IN CONCLUSION

It is more than likely that toxemia and subsequent pathology result from the absorption of certain chemicals formed by the bacterial action on certain amino acids. Alexis Carrel, M.D., a noted French surgeon and winner of the Nobel Prize for physiology and medicine in 1912, clearly demonstrated the relationship in an experiment involving the hearts of chicken embryos. The French-born physician and biochemist was working at the Rockefeller Institute for Medical Research in New York when he placed microslices of heart tissue from a chicken embryo on microscope slides and performed one of the most remarkable experiments in medical history. He attempted to demonstrate that under suitable conditions, the living cell could survive for a very long time, perhaps indefinitely.

The tissues on the slides were rinsed daily in a solution from which they obtained the necessary nutrients and in which they deposited their wastes. Every day, the solution was changed. It is amazing to report that these tissue cells survived for twenty-nine years in this fashion. They died one day only because the laboratory assistant neglected to rinse them with fresh nutrient solution. In other words, autointoxication claimed this great masterpiece of experimental scientific investigation. Said Dr. Carrel of this experience, "The cell is immortal. It is merely the fluid in which it floats which degenerates. Renew this fluid at intervals, give the cell something upon which to feed and, so far as we know, the pulsation of life may go on forever." Dr. Carrel's experiment is just one example of how putrefactive waste products cause pathological conditions.

"Pathology" is classically defined as "abnormal function." The doctors discussed earlier in this chapter demonstrated that there is a clinical, clearly observable relationship between intestinal toxemia and abnormal cellular function. Their reports reveal thousands of cases in which people suffering from various ills improved or became well after clearing up their intestinal toxemia. For example, eczema is a pathological change, and it was healed time and again when the source of the irritation—intestinal toxemia—was removed. In a clinical discussion, it is highly relevant and important to note that many sick people have become well when their intestinal toxemia was cleared up. On the other hand, medical opinion holds that the causes of conditions such as Crohn's disease, Whipple's disease, and ulcerative colitis are unknown. But the irritation that causes the primary inflammation in these afflictions must come from somewhere, or the science of pathology must re-examine its basic assumptions.

After years of work in nutrition and colon cleansing, I cannot help but conclude that the symptoms of many chronic diseases are directly or indirectly associated with intestinal putrefaction. In light of my clinical experience, I can draw no other conclusion.

Chapter 3

Common Bowel Disorders

G astrointestinal disorders abound. More people are admitted to hospitals with digestive complaints than any other malady. Although it seems "nicer" to speak of digestive disorders than bowel disorders, we must not forget that the gastrointestinal tract is but a single system from the mouth to the anus and includes the stomach and bowel.

In addition to diet, one of the primary influences upon the bowel is emotional strain. Any emotional strain on the body affects the intestinal tract. In fact, the intestinal tract also influences the emotions. It is common in our society to speak of the emotions as being associated with the heart. People who are emotionally upset or under tension may indeed suffer heart problems, but they are much more likely to suffer intestinal distress such as gastritis, heartburn, ulcers, colitis, irritable bowel syndrome, constipation, or diarrhea, to name but a few.

Nervous tension causes contractions in all the orifices of the body. People under stress and strain have contracted pupils. When we learn to let go of the negatives, the pupils of our eyes relax, as do the muscles around the anus and other orifices. If the anus is contracted at the time of elimination, it is difficult to get rid of all the toxic material in the rectum. As with all nervous and mental tensions, the cause must be dealt with before any lasting relief can be achieved in regard to strictures (abnormal narrowing) in the bowel.

The stomach, the seat of much gastric distress, is merely a distention of the gut tube, a temporary holding pouch for food, and the site of the preliminary stages of digestion. Some so-called stomach distur-

45

bances are actually the result of problems that lie further down the intestinal tract. An analogy is a kitchen sink backing up. The cause of the problem often is not the sink itself, but rather an obstruction down in the pipe.

Although people complain of a host of digestive problems, many of their complaints can be traced to the bowel. Some of their complaints can even be traced specifically to constipation. Stomach troubles include deficiencies of pepsin and hydrochloric acid, while bowel problems range from variable transit time for waste to inadequate bile secretion. The most common bowel problem by far is constipation.

CONSTIPATION

Up to this point, we have raised our bowel consciousness to include knowledge of the effects of intestinal toxemia and autointoxication. We should now give consideration to the bowel condition that affects more people than all the other colon complaints combined. So universal is this condition that virtually everyone experiences it. Some have only fleeting episodes. Many more suffer on a frequent or even continual basis, reaping the consequences of the condition's long-term toxic effects. I am referring to constipation.

We will come to see that constipation is much more than a simple and temporary failure or a chronic difficulty in having a bowel movement. Bowel difficulties such as constipation and its resultant autointoxication, which are symptoms of a poor diet and lifestyle, cause a multitude of evils that are ruinous in their consequences. I am beginning this chapter with a discussion of constipation because nearly all of the bowel disorders considered in this book are associated with it in some way.

Constipation is often referred to by those who have studied it as the "modern plague." Indeed, I consider it the greatest present-day internal danger to health. Intestinal toxemia and autointoxication are direct results of intestinal constipation. Constipation contributes to the lowering of the body's resistance, predisposing the body to many acute illnesses and the initiation of many degenerative and chronic processes. Constipation indirectly cripples and kills more people in our country than almost any other single disease condition having to do with deficient function.

Constipation also increases the workload of the other excretory organs—the skin, the kidneys, the lymphatic system, and the lungs. These other organs and systems become hyperactive, overworked, and eventually worn out. Cellular metabolism thus becomes sluggish, repair and growth delayed, the ability to eliminate waste materials compromised, and the body less energetic. The cells, instead of being alive and vibrant, become inactive and dull. The result is a decline in functional ability, beginning with the physiologically weakest organs, glands, tissues, and systems of the body.

Bowel movements every two to three days are considered normal by many people and even by some medical doctors. I believe otherwise. My experiences have proven beyond a doubt that inadequate bowel movements and poor bowel hygiene (resulting in autointoxication) are the sources of an untold number of disorders in the body. We must be mindful of the difference between what is considered normal and what is correct or desirable from a health standpoint.

Constipation is so widespread that the average person who is constipated doesn't even know it. Physicians, depending on their specialty, may think of the frequency of "normal" bowel movements as being anything from two to fourteen times per week. People from primitive cultures who live totally apart from modern civilization and consume a diet of pure, whole, natural foods—foods unprocessed and seldom cooked—usually have a bowel movement about one-half hour following each meal. Westerners who consume many processed and devitalized foods, usually cooked or even overcooked, are happy to attain one bowel movement a day. So you see, defining what is correct and exactly what constitutes constipation is not such an easy task. Our lifestyles, both personally and as a society in general, have to be considered in any determination of the correct number and timing of bowel movements.

We have to stop and think that when we eat, peristaltic action in the bowel moves the food and its residue down to the last part of the elimination system, the large intestine. Normally, it takes eighteen hours for food to go through the body and be eliminated. The time it takes for ingested food to travel the length of the intestinal tract and be ready for elimination is known as bowel transit time. Transit time is less when we eat a diet rich in bulk and indigestible fiber, and also get adequate amounts of fresh air, sunshine, water, and exercise. On the other hand, when people live indoors; eat fiber-deficient, cooked, and processed foods; and are generally sedentary, bowel transit time is slowed. More than anything else, the extra time that food residues remain in the intestine contributes to the formation of toxic substances, alters intestinal flora, and results in intestinal toxemia and autointoxication. Some people have only one bowel movement a week, and others two bowel movements a week. I had a patient who had a bowel movement every eighteen days and still consumed three meals a day. Assuming we eat three meals a day and have a bowel movement once every five days, we're fourteen meals behind. Figure 3.1 shows how food moves through the gastrointestinal tract in a twenty-four-hour period and what happens when the bowel doesn't eliminate on time.

However, the frequency of fecal elimination is not the sole indication of constipation or regularity. It is common for people to think of diarrhea as being the opposite of constipation. In fact, diarrhea is usually just another form of constipation. When the bowel becomes impacted with feces, the body will often liquefy the colon contents in a last-ditch effort to rid itself of the toxic-waste accumulation. Continued diarrhea can severely dehydrate the body and upset its electrolyte balance. The first thing people usually do is take an over-the-counter preparation to stop the diarrhea while remaining unaware that the condition may be a sign of constipation. When diarrhea of this kind is suppressed, the constipation and its causes remain unattended.

Some of my patients believe that if they have three bowel movements a day, they have diarrhea, while others think that a couple of movements a week is normal. An example of the latter was a patient who assured me that she had normal bowel movements. She related that her bowel moved regularly every Tuesday and Friday morning! I know of people who had three or four movements a day and yet the bowel wall was quite encrusted and the bowel itself was very constipated.

Most people do not know the condition of their bowel. Unfortunately, those who are not aware of their bowel function or condition are sometimes the ones who develop the worst bowel troubles. Most people were not properly educated in childhood to realize the importance of adequate daily elimination and to heed nature's call to evacuate the bowel. This indifference to the natural urge to evacuate the bowel may be the cause of the beginning of constipation.

Both British and South African medical scientists strongly insist that what is usually referred to as regularity may be a matter of life and death. Insufficient numbers of bowel movements and too little fiber and bulk in the feces may often explain the existence of gallbladder disorders, heart problems, varicose veins, appendicitis, clotting in the deep veins, hiatal hernia, diverticulosis, arthritis, and cancer of the colon. This complete turn-around in medical orientation comes from top-notch medical researchers such as Dr. Denis Burkitt. (See "Denis P. Burkitt, M.D." on page 52.)

John Harvey Kellogg, M.D., of the famous Battle Creek

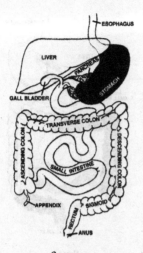

8 A.M.

The shaded area shows the food in the stomach immediately after breakfast.

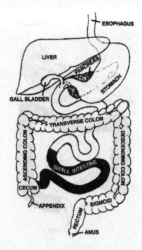

Noon.

Four hours after breakfast, the food has reached the ileum and ileocecal valve. Digestion and absorption are completed, and the unused residue of breakfast is ready to be passed into the colon.

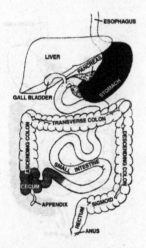

1 P.M.

The lightly shaded area shows the breakfast residue passing through the ileocecal valve into the colon. The dark shading shows lunch in the stomach.

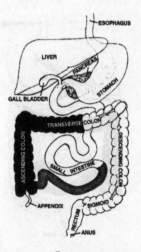

5 P.M.

The lightly shaded area shows the breakfast residue in the colon. The dark area shows the lunch residue ready to enter the colon.

Figure 3.1. How food is ingested and travels through the intestinal tract.

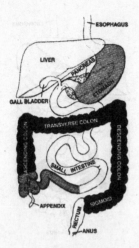

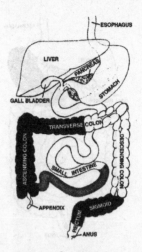

6 P.M.

The lightly shaded area shows the break-fast residue mostly in the descending colon. The lunch residue is passing into the colon and mixing with the breakfast residue. The dark area shows dinner just eaten and in the stomach.

9 P.M.

The breakfast residue is in the sigmoid colon, ready to be discharged. The lunch residue is in the cecum and the ascending and transverse colon. The dinner residue is ready to enter the colon.

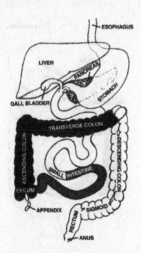

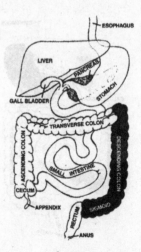

10 P.M.

The breakfast residue has been discharged via a bowel movement at bedtime. The lunch residue is moving through the colon. The dinner residue is waiting to enter the colon.

6 A.M.

The dinner residue is in the descending and sigmoid colon, ready to be dis-charged.

Figure 3.1 continued

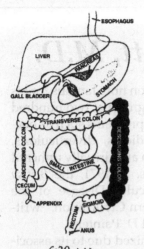

6:30 A.M.
A bowel movement has just occurred. The residue of the previous night's dinner is left in the colon.

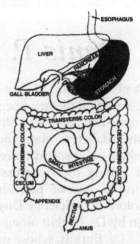

8 A.M.
The bowel has completely evacuated in preparation for a new series of meals. Breakfast is in the stomach.

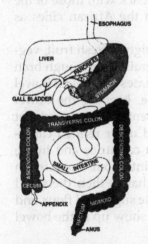

If the bowel is moved only once a day, it will contain the residue of six meals.

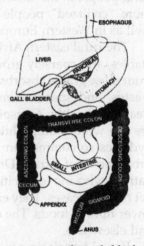

If nine or more meals are held, chronic constipation will exists.

Sanitarium in Battle Creek, Michigan, did more work in connection with intestinal sanitation than anyone else in the United States. He lived to be ninety-one. His advice is worth listening to. He believed that we should eliminate the residue of each meal fifteen to eighteen hours after consuming the meal. Babies, birds, and animals evacuate

Denis P. Burkitt, M.D.

Denis P. Burkitt, M.D., a British surgeon now famous for his research on dietary fiber, once told a group of two hundred prominent American physicians that problems such as obesity, diabetes, hiatal hernia, appendicitis, diverticulosis, colitis, polyps, and cancer of the colon are virtually unheard of among the rural eastern Africans. In 1971, the *British Medical Journal* published "Diverticular Disease of the Colon: A Deficiency Disease of Western Civilization," written by Dr. Burkitt along with Dr. Neil D. Painter.

Dr. Burkitt, whose name is recognized due to its association with Burkitt's lymphoma, a specific type of cancer, spent most of his adult life at Makerere University and Mulago Hospital in Kampala, Uganda, where he had the opportunity to compare the health and dietary habits of the rural people in the eastern Africa outback with those of the more "civilized" people dwelling in the African cities as well as in Western Europe.

The rural eastern African diet is high in fresh fruit, vegetables, and coarsely ground cereal grains. The rough bran from these grains absorbs water, increases the bulk of bowel wastes, and speeds elimination time, keeping the bowel clean and healthy. Conspicuously absent from the rural diet are the white flour, white sugar, and other refined carbohydrates so common in the Western countries and in the urban areas of Africa. Dr. Burkitt pointed out that African natives who move to cities tend to change their diets and get more diseases. They eat more white sugar and flour, and fewer fibrous foods. The effects soon show up in the bowel and elsewhere.

Bowel transit time in a Bantu native is more than twice that of the average Englishman, according to Dr. Burkitt's research. This is because the native's average daily intake of fiber is about 100 milligrams, as opposed to less than half that amount for the "more civilized" individual. The length of time food wastes remain in the bowel determines how putrefactive they become, how much the undesirable bacteria multiply, how much fat is absorbed through the bowel wall, and what sort of chemical toxins develop in and pass through the bowel.

Based on the data he gathered in the Congo, Kenya, Uganda, Sudan, and other underdeveloped parts of the world, Dr. Burkitt became a proponent of proper bowel care through correct nutrition. He said that diet, especially one in which there is an increase in dietary fiber and a reduction in processed, fiber-depleted carbohydrates, is the key to preventing much disease and needless surgery. He believes that the overconsumption of refined, fiber-depleted carbohydrates is responsible for arteriosclerosis and diabetes, and that the absence of sufficient fiber in the diet promotes colon diseases. Excessive consumption of refined carbohydrates favors the growth of putrefactive bacteria in the bowel, alters bowel chemistry, and invites ulcerative colitis, polyps, and colon cancer. After Dr. Burkitt extended his research to include diseases other than those of the bowel, he coauthored "Dietary Fiber and Disease," again with Dr. Painter. This article appeared in the August 19, 1974, issue of the *Journal of the American Medical Association*.

much sooner after a meal. I heard Dr. Kellogg say that he knew of many cases in which operations were avoided because the bowel was cleansed and revitalized. He maintained that 90 percent of the diseases of civilization are due to improper functioning of the colon. Dr. Lane also pointed out the relationship between intestinal toxemia and disease. He left no doubt as to how seriously he regarded the effects of intestinal intoxication when he said, "The lower end of the intestine is of the size that requires emptying every six hours, but by habit we retain its contents twenty-four hours. The result is ulcers and cancer."

Constipation, whatever its form, always results in a clogging of the colon. This clogging occurs in several ways. A primary way is mucous buildup on the irritated mucous membrane and bowel wall to such an extent that feces can hardly pass through. One autopsy revealed a distended colon that was nine inches in diameter but had a passageway through it no larger than the diameter of a common wood pencil! The rest was layer upon layer of encrusted mucus and fecal material. Mucus accumulation can have the consistency of hard rubber not unlike that of an automobile tire. Another autopsy revealed a stagnant colon that weighed an incredible forty pounds! Imagine carrying around all that morbid accumulated waste. The need for bowel sanitation and cleanliness has been sadly neglected by nearly everyone.

I am convinced that the bowel holds on to waste material longer than anyone realizes. When we clean the bowel and release all this old, rotting material, gas, pain, and autointoxication are lessened. I believe that the toxic material decaying in the sigmoid colon provides a favorable environment for the onset of degenerative disease.

What, then, is required to move the bowel contents along on time? Good bowel tone gives the intestinal tract the power to move waste materials properly through the system. Good tone is developed and maintained by following a proper diet and getting enough exercise. Diets rich in fiber are required to give the intestinal musculature something to work against. Consider how weight lifters use weights to give their muscles something to work against. Strength and tone cannot be developed or maintained unless there is opposition to muscular action. Dietary bulk provides indigestible material for the intestinal muscles to "work against." In like manner, exercising the trunk, especially the abdominal wall and back, helps keep the intestine in its proper place and provides structures with good tone for the intestine to work against. Most primitive cultures have dance movements that exercise the trunk, back, and abdominal muscles. Modern Westerners, on the contrary, dance with their legs, and they do this almost to the exclusion of using the trunk, upper extremities, and neck. With proper diet and exercise, the intestine can work against good muscle tone externally and against resistant bulky fiber material internally.

Poor habits contribute a great deal to functional constipation, which is not caused by developmental abnormalities or associated with any disease. It may lead to structural problems or disease, however, if not corrected. Failure to follow a good daily regimen denies the body regularity and consistency. People who have busy schedules often eat sketchy meals, and those meals only if and when they have time. They do not set aside regular periods for sitting at stool, or for resting, sleeping, and exercising. With this lifestyle, the body never knows what's coming next. It is always on the defensive. The result is a depletion of vital energy and another step toward bowel irregularity and constipation.

Most people do not drink enough water to help ensure proper bowel function. Insufficient liquid in the diet causes chronic dehydration and can be one of the major contributing factors to constipation.

Lack of moisture reduces the volume of all the bodily fluids and thickens some of them. The bodily tissues become drier and less functional. The mucous lining in the colon changes in consistency, failing to provide slick lubrication for the movement of feces.

Other factors such as the underactivity of the other elimination organs may contribute to constipation. Enough bile must come from the gallbladder and the liver to emulsify fats and help give the bowel its natural incentive to produce bowel movements. In addition, the thyroid gland, which is important in controlling the body's metabolic rate, must function properly. The thyroid regulates a number of functions and keeps them normal by releasing the hormone thyroxin into the body. When the thyroid is underactive, all the bodily functions are slowed. Slowed digestion can lead to constipation.

If the adrenal glands are underactive, a person can feel so tired and fatigued that he or she doesn't feel up to exercising. Both fatigue and lack of exercise promote constipation. You have to feel lively to get going and move. Another condition that produces fatigue is anemia, which can keep you from a healthy level of physical activity. If your blood is anemic, it has insufficient oxygen, and your bodily tissues produce less energy. You are "tired all over," so to speak. A tired body cannot eliminate well.

The Laxative Debacle

Many people spend a good deal of money trying to overcome or avoid constipation. If, for instance, the bowel lacks sufficient tone to move its contents satisfactorily, we turn to laxatives. Roughly 95 percent of all laxatives are irritating to the bowel, forcing peristaltic action by means of this irritation.

There are said to be more than 45,000 laxative and cathartic remedies manufactured and used in the United States alone. In a recent year, laxative sales were conservatively placed at $350 million. That's a lot of constipation! Even when used sparingly and just in emergencies, laxatives should be approached with great caution. The mechanism of elimination is very delicate and easily upset. Once disturbed, it often requires weeks, maybe months, to become regular again. Laxatives, in order to evacuate the colon, are essentially poisons and irritants. They contribute nothing to the restoration of the normal or natural process of defecation. The poisoned colon tries to evacuate the offending substance as quickly as possible, and pushes everything out, including the compacted feces.

Oftentimes, these harsh poisonous substances are absorbed into the lymph and blood vessels, and find their way to all the parts of the body. This situation contributes to the addiction and overuse of laxatives. Dependency upon laxative compounds over time permanently destroys the normal ability of the bowel to eliminate of its own accord. Laxatives tire out the bowel muscle by keeping it constantly working. Without rest, the muscle soon fails and produces some of the conditions discussed later in this chapter. The only stimulation the bowel should have is from exercise, normal nerve impulses, and proper diet. Any time the bowel is artificially stimulated, an undesirable result is a loss of muscle tone, eventually producing a weakness in that muscle structure.

DIVERTICULAR DISEASE

Constipation is not the only colon condition that is prevalent in Western cultures. Having bowel pockets, properly called diverticula, is not the least unusual. Those who have them are said to have diverticular disease of the colon, more commonly called diverticulosis.

Diverticula constitute a deviation of the normal and regular bowel wall. In cases of faulty bowel elimination, diverticula, which resemble little sacs, form along the wall of the large intestine. (See Figure 3.2, below.) Diverticula may also form in the esophagus, stomach, duodenum, and jejunum (the section of the small intestine immediately following the duodenum and extending to the ileum). A single diverticulum may also form in the cecum or elsewhere in the colon.

Diverticulosis and diverticulitis many times cause confusion. Often these terms are used interchangeably and wrongly. We must be clear about their definitions. The words "diverticulosis" and "diverti-

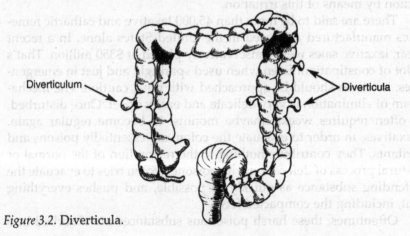

Diverticulum

Diverticula

Figure 3.2. Diverticula.

culitis" have the common Latin root of *divertu*, which means "to turn aside." Diverticulosis, as mentioned, refers to pockets protruding from the bowel wall. Although these diverticula may cause no direct symptoms, they can sometimes be the source of troubles elsewhere in the body, as we shall see later. Diverticular disease of the colon can be a serious disturbance leading to many difficulties. Therefore, it must be prevented or controlled. If the diverticula become inflamed, the condition is called diverticulitis. The suffix "-itis" refers to an inflammation. When inflamed diverticula become infected, it is a serious condition known as acute diverticulitis, which requires immediate professional attention. We should be aware that the complications of diverticulitis can carry a high price tag. Death is not unheard of in the advanced stages, and a vast amount of chronic ill health and symptomatology are evident in the early stages. Bowel pockets need not become inflamed if cared for properly. Although many people have diverticulosis, only a relatively small number develop acute diverticulitis.

Diverticula and the Sigmoid Colon

Diverticula are found in the sigmoid colon more often than in any other area of the bowel. In a British study, sigmoid diverticula were found in 443 out of 461 cases of diverticulosis. In a study by Dr. L.E. Hughes in Australia, 89 of 90 diseased colons had diverticula in the sigmoid. Dr. Hughes believes that this high incidence of diverticulosis in the sigmoid colon is due to this part of the colon being so narrow. Because of its small diameter, the sigmoid harbors the firmest feces and produces the highest degree of colonic pressure.

When the diet is deficient in bulk or fiber, the colonic muscles must work extremely hard to force the feces through the lower bowel. Where there is a weakness in the muscle fibers, a hernia can occur, producing a diverticulum in the bowel wall. A hernia resembles the blister that occurs on the side wall of an automobile tire when air is forced to a part of the surface where the wall has thinned.

Diverticula tend to retain some fecal waste as it passes by, very much like the pockets in a meandering stream that catch and retain flotsam from the main current. As time passes, these diverticula accumulate more and more waste matter. When the bowel is sluggish and transit time increased, conditions occur that can cause infection due to the prolonged contact between the accumulated material and the diverticula. The diverticula then become seedbeds for the production of powerful toxins, adding to an already overburdened and toxic body. When this happens, there is immediate autointoxication and a danger of septicemia (blood-borne infection).

If the infected diverticula rupture, bacteria and toxic wastes spew into the abdominal cavity, causing acute peritonitis (inflammation of the abdominal cavity's lining). When this occurs, it is an immediate medical and surgical emergency. Often, a colostomy must be performed. In a colostomy, the colon is surgically severed and brought to an opening in the surface of the skin to allow the feces to pass through the patient's side directly into a bag. If the colon is in such bad shape that some or all of it must be removed, the procedure is called a colectomy. In a large number of colostomies, at least a portion of the colon is removed. This portion is often pocketed with inflamed, infected, or ruptured diverticula that are life-threatening to the patient. Colostomies and other types of surgical intervention are sometimes considered the only methods that can prevent further colon complications and allow the patient to live a more or less normal life.

Many adverse conditions develop long before surgery is even considered as an option. Because the sigmoid colon always contains the driest part of the stool, it has to withstand the greatest amount of pressure in trying to get rid of the stool. It is here that the driest fecal material works the greatest hardship on the mucosa of the bowel wall.

I believe it is the action of increased pressure on inherently weaker portions of the bowel wall that contributes the most to the development of diverticula. This pressure can be associated with a sedentary job or lifestyle, legs that are crossed or bent throughout the day, and a thickening of the circular and longitudinal muscles of the colon. Furthermore, due to the faulty design of the modern toilet, there is a greater strain on the sigmoid than on any other part of the intestinal tract. (See "Complications of the Modern Toilet" on page 150.) These conditions each make a preclinical contribution to the disease, but I believe that a genetic or constitutional weakness in the bowel is the most significant risk factor for diverticular disease of the colon.

My experience and research have led me to the belief that the origin of diverticular disease is in the embryo. It is my conclusion that people are born with weak spots in the structure of their bowel walls. As life progresses, the bowel wall is taxed, stressed, and weakened by bad habits. The genetically weaker areas of the bowel cannot stand up to the constant abuse and thus develop disorders such as diverticular disease. Many doctors today call this condition leaky bowel syndrome. (See "Leaky Bowel Syndrome" on page 59.)

Researchers are finding that an ever-increasing number of young people have colon diverticula. Diverticular disease of the colon used

Leaky Bowel Syndrome

A condition called leaky bowel syndrome is currently getting a lot of attention from the various healing professions. Leaky bowel syndrome includes the various problems that result from the "leakage" of undesirable materials through the bowel wall into the blood and lymph. I have been writing and lecturing about this syndrome for over forty years. However, I didn't give the condition a name, and I describe it a little differently. I believe that leaky bowel syndrome is a result of what I have for some time been calling "inherent weakness."

Many years ago, I recognized that harmful lifestyle habits together with inherent weaknesses can cause changes in the bowel that allow the absorption of toxic materials through the bowel wall. These harmful lifestyle habits include deficient diet, lack of exercise, and poor bowel habits. By "inherent weaknesses," I mean inherently weak (defective) tissue that lacks the strength and integrity of normal tissue. We might compare normal tissue to silk and inherently weak tissue to burlap. Burlap is so coarsely woven that it can't hold liquids the way silk can. Inherently weak tissue assimilates nutrients poorly, eliminates metabolic wastes more slowly, and is more prone to inflammation than normal tissue. It is more easily broken down. It is more subject to disease.

Inherent weaknesses in the bowel in time may show up as ballooning, diverticula, spasm, slowed transit time, or any of a number of diseases. It is my experience that many health disorders and diseases begin with problems in the elimination system. Leaky bowel syndrome kicks off with any of the basic conditions I just mentioned.

As far as I am concerned, leaky bowel syndrome is not new. In the 1930s, I was working with Dr. Glen Sipes when he visited a patient burning up with fever. The patient's skin was beet red, and he was in great pain. His problem was severe constipation. Dr. Sipes treated him with enemas, and the man was soon resting comfortably. His fever and redness disappeared. I believe Dr. Sipes removed the cause of the problem when he cleansed the patient's bowel and stopped the "leakage" of toxins into the blood and lymph.

Where do inherent weaknesses in the bowel come from? We have found that the genetic strengths and weaknesses of the parents show up early in the development of the embryo. As the fertilized cell begins to grow and mature inside the mother, the bowel is formed before any of the other organs. Next, tiny buds that will later become the limbs and internal organs appear on the bowel. The bowel tissue covering these buds eventually becomes the exterior membrane covering the organs that develop from the buds. Because of this, the relationship between the bowel and the internal organs of the body is an ongoing one. Furthermore, if the embryonic bowel had an area of inherent weakness, and this area of inherent weakness had a bud form and grow, then the organ that developed from that bud will have that inherent weaknesses. This means that toxic material from an inherently weak area of the bowel can migrate to the tissue in an internal organ that was related to that part of the bowel during the embryonic stage of development. This is why I consider leaky bowel syndrome to be very important.

I feel that one of my greatest discoveries is how a certain place in the bowel can affect a certain organ. I call this the neural-arc reflex. (For a full discussion of the neural-arc reflex, see Chapter 4.) The concept of the neural-arc reflex was once again clearly reinforced for me during a recent trip to Florida. In Florida, I visited a friend who had recently had a slight heart attack. I had warned my friend that his bowel problems could cause him heart trouble. Now, when my friend feels pain in the area of his descending colon, he immediately takes a colema. This is because the descending colon has a reflex relationship with the heart. It is to our advantage to take care of the bowel to prevent the migration of toxic materials from inherently weak areas in the bowel to the corresponding inherently weak areas in the internal organs by means of this reflex relationship.

Leaky bowel syndrome always indicates a need for bowel cleansing and for appropriate changes in the diet and lifestyle. I always take care of the bowel first, no matter what symptoms I find in other organs.

I first learned about the relationship between the bowel and the rest of the body from Max Gerson, M.D. Dr. Gerson refused to allow his patients to depend on pain medication. If a patient complained of pain, he prescribed an enema. The pain invariably left. From the holistic viewpoint, we can't treat just an organ. We have to treat the whole person. We have to get to the root of the problem. When we take care of the bowel, we take care of the whole body.

It is to our advantage to take care of a leaky bowel as soon as we notice any symptoms. The best way to prevent the neural-arc reflex from causing symptoms in internal organs is to do a thorough cleansing of the bowel. Inherent weaknesses themselves are not dangerous. They are nothing more than areas of weakness. If we live in harmony with nature—eating right, breathing clean fresh air, getting enough rest, exercising every day, thinking positive thoughts, enjoying beauty, existing at peace with God and man—we could live forever with our inherent weaknesses. This, I feel, is a goal worth working for.

to be considered a condition of advanced age. I believe it is being seen regularly in ever-younger people due to the kinds of foods children eat, as well as fail to eat, today. The effects of poor nutrition are being seen in the genetically weaker areas of the body at earlier ages. G.G. Turner, in 1920, and L.A. Buie, in 1939, were among the first to postulate the congenital factor in diverticulosis. Buie also predicted an increase in childhood diverticulosis. Unfortunately, he has been proven correct.

There are some researchers who do not agree that diverticula are genetically predisposed. Researchers Conell, Riley, and Painter concluded that colonic diverticulitis is not due to a congenital weakness. Rather, they stated, the colonic muscle is normal at birth and changes only in later years. But how could they tell that there was no congenital weakness at birth? A congenital weakness cannot be X-rayed or determined except through a system of analysis that can detect such specific inherent tissue weaknesses. The orthodox medicine of today has no such system and rejects traditional alternative health practices that may include one.

A genetic weakness can be exacerbated by bad habits that promote faulty elimination and increased gas pressure. These include eating gas-forming foods, neglecting to set aside regular times for bowel evacuation, straining to pass hard stools, and living a fast-paced, stressful lifestyle accompanied by faulty nutrition.

The role of diet in controlling diverticulosis was first postulated by Dr. Neil S. Painter, a fellow of the Royal College of Surgeons in England, and Dr. Denis Burkitt. When these two men began their research, they erroneously believed that because of intracolonic pressure in patients with diverticulosis, a low-residue (minimal-fiber) diet was the indicated nutritional treatment. Later, as the research continued, the doctors became convinced that this was not the case. They found that a minimal-fiber diet causes more gas and pressure during elimination and that surgical attempts at correction sometimes complicate the problem. By introducing oat bran into the diets of their London patients and observing a significant reduction in symptoms, including intracolonic pressure, the doctors determined that a high-fiber diet is more beneficial. This led them to draw several important conclusions that are at the core of much of our current treatment.

At the Mayo Clinic in the 1930s, doctors began to compare the effects on the sigmoid colon of a low-residue diet versus a high-fiber diet. They found that fiber prevents the bowel from becoming flaccid and lazy. Natural, pure, and whole foods can help to develop bowel tone. Proper diet was thus introduced as a viable alternative to surgery.

Diverticular disease isn't a matter of not having enough fiber in the diet for just one or two days. It's a matter of neglecting to have it over a period of many years. Fast and inharmonious living, not chewing food properly, patronizing fast-food restaurants, eating foods that lack natural fiber, and removing or not eating the skin from vegetables and fruits deprive the bowel of adequate bulk and moisture retention. In eliminating the natural fiber that we should have, we deprive the bowel wall of material to exercise against. When the diet lacks bulk or fiber, the colonic muscle must work extremely hard to force the drier feces through the colon. Without this natural exercise function, increased intraluminal (within the gut tube) pressures cause diverticula to form in the inherently weaker sections of the bowel wall.

In the United States, with all our refined, highly processed, over-cooked foods, we have a higher incidence of bowel disease than is found in countries where a high-fiber diet is the norm. Consider the native African diet, which is high in fiber and devoid of overcooked and processed foods. Diverticular disease is almost unknown in Africa. However, when the natives become habituated to a Western diet, the frequency of the disease rises. In fact, diverticular disease of the colon is virtually unknown in any of the so-called primitive societies that eat from the natural bounty of the land. Studies have shown that people living under primitive conditions on diets high in indigestible fiber pass from two-and-a-half to four-and-a-half times as much feces as people in modern Western civilizations. Those studies revealed that diverticular disease of the colon appears to be directly related to a high-carbohydrate, low-fiber diet such as one containing denatured white flour and processed sugar.

Although it is a corrective move to add more fiber to the diet, people who change quickly from a smooth diet of pancakes, pasta, and many of the other soft foods we have today to one of extreme roughage occasionally experience bowel disturbances. Sometimes, the increase in gas and other bowel disturbances can make a person have second thoughts about whether to change the diet! The problem here is that the body does not adapt rapidly to extreme changes. This situation can usually be minimized, if not avoided, by making the change to a higher fiber intake over a more extended period. The gradual introduction of more roughage into the diet allows the body to slowly make the necessary changes to accommodate the new diet.

If genetic weaknesses can be determined to exist in a person, four lifestyle changes can help to prevent the manifestation of diverticulosis. They are as follows:

1. Reducing the pressure from gases associated with imbalance in the intestinal flora.

2. Answering nature's call on demand.

3. Squatting to avoid the pressure on the anus and sigmoid colon created by the use of the modern toilet.

4. Holding the hands above the head while bearing down on the toilet to avoid exerting force against the delicate rectal tissues. (See "Ileocecal-Valve Dysfunction" on page 152.)

It is sad that we do not raise our children to realize that having a bowel movement is the most important bodily function. Even as adults, we often get too busy and let things slide. We put aside care of the bowel for later. We often believe that we cannot take care of it now—but later may be too late. Many specialists today conclude that, like the rest of the body, the colon becomes more susceptible to diverticular and other diseases as a result of the aging process. To take this one step further, I believe that the years of extra pressure acting upon the sigmoid colon also contribute to certain types of heart troubles and may even mimic some heart-attack symptoms, such as pain in the chest and left arm, which more often emerge in the middle and later years.

Diverticular disease of the colon is occurring at an ever-increasing rate. As a result of research done in the past twenty-five years, we now know a great deal about the disease. Many studies in addition to the one by Dr. Hughes have been done on the various aspects of diverticulosis. Dr. Harold Edwards discovered that when the circular muscle of the colon is thickened and internal pressure is increased, the function of the bowel becomes inhibited. Though this muscle in this condition first appears to be strong, closer inspection reveals that the thickening actually consists of groups of muscle fibers bundled together with gaps in the structure of the muscle itself. Dr. Edwards thinks this situation might also account for episodes of acute pain and tenderness, transient fever, and a large increase in the number of nucleated white blood cells.

The best way to find out if diverticula are present is with a barium enema. This procedure should always include two X-ray series— one when the bowel is full of the barium meal and one after it has been emptied. Years ago, I was astonished by the results of one patient's X-rays. The first series revealed some of the barium meal remaining in little diverticula. A week later, another X-ray was taken of the same patient as part of a gallbladder series. In the new X-rays, I was able to see some barium still settled in various diverticula throughout the colon. If a barium meal can stay in the colon for a week, cannot fecal material also stay there? No material should remain in the colon for a week's time!

In Dr. Edwards' study of 179 barium-enema patients, 91 percent of the patients had diverticular disease. In 95 of these patients, only the sigmoid colon was diseased; 38 patients had sigmoid and descending colons with diverticula; 18 had sigmoid, descending, and transverse colons that were affected; and 13 had entire colons that were beset with diverticula.

Health practitioners need to develop a program whereby diverticula can be detected even before they show up on X-ray examination or become a waiting-room complaint. We need to understand, too, that whenever there is a genetic weakness in the bowel that predisposes a person to diverticulosis, there is also a great probability of genetic weakness in other areas of the body. We then must apply the proper bowel regimen, including the establishment of correct living habits, in order to minimize the chances of the formation of diverticula. When diverticula are found to be present, we need to know how to take care of the entire bowel.

COLITIS

Colitis is an irritable bowel condition that is often associated with psychological distress. "Colitis" means "inflammation of the colon." People who suffer from colitis may have constipation alternating with bouts of bloody diarrhea, abdominal cramps, high fever, and malaise. A person may have from fifteen to twenty-five watery bowel movements a day with no relief, even during the nighttime hours. They may also have a loss of appetite with a corresponding weight loss.

Although a colitis condition may be partially associated with the wrong diet or with genetic weaknesses that make the bowel more prone to manifest this disease, it is nearly always associated with, or brought on by, a psychological condition. Few people truly realize the benefits of a calm and peaceful lifestyle. They are often unaware of the mind's ability to influence the body's function. Fear, anger, depression, stress, tension, worries, and obsessions can all upset the delicate processes of the body, in particular those of digestion and elimination. The same as most other disorders, colitis is best treated by removing the cause—that is, the causes of the stress and neurosis should be determined and removed, if possible. Sometimes, what we need is a good cerebral laxative to rid the mind of emotional autointoxication and constipation. In addition, necessary and appropriate changes should be made in the diet and lifestyle.

In acute episodes of ulcerative colitis, the colon may be in such an irritated state that only a liquid diet can be tolerated. Soothing mucilaginous drinks, such as flaxseed tea, may be sipped. High-quality, nonirritating foods, mainly fruits and vegetables, should be liquefied in a blender and drunk. When the inflammation subsides, a nonirritating bulk such as psyllium can be introduced. Liquid chlorophyll is a good dietary additive to promote healing of the inflamed areas. In all cases, we must be aware that colitis is a dangerous condition and requires the expert attention of a qualified health practitioner.

Medical solutions for irritated portions of the colon include antiinflammatory medications, colostomy, and often colectomy. Sometimes a colostomy is temporary, performed to give the irritated portion of the colon a rest. According to the National Center for Health Statistics, every year 57,000 people in the United States undergo colostomies, certainly a radical procedure.

Inflammatory colon problems such a colitis, ileitis, and diverticulitis affect, by conservative estimates, 2,000,000 people in the United States. Medical professionals admit that although decades of research have been conducted on these diseases, the cures remain elusive.

STRICTURE

A stricture of the bowel usually occurs after an inflammatory disease such as colitis has damaged the bowel tissue. A chronic narrowing of the intestinal passageway, stricture often results in a backup of feces unable to pass through the narrowed lumen. The feces accumulate in front of the stricture, causing ballooning of the colon, while the segment just past the stricture collapses, as seen in Figure 3.3. The stricture creates a bottleneck that makes the passage of fecal material difficult. Only when the pinched area becomes relaxed can fecal material pass more or less freely.

Some strictures are more severe than others. Strictures may be caused by a long-term flow of aberrant nerve impulses to a particular area of the colon, often as a result of stress or stress-associated conditions. If the condition persists long enough, a nervous pathway is established. Thus, it becomes increasingly easier for nerve impulses to take this particular route. In addition, there may be an inherent weakness in a certain area of the bowel that also serves to facilitate the formation of a stricture. Intestinal strictures may be associated with

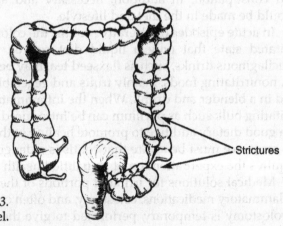

Strictures

Figure 3.3.
Strictures of the bowel.

inherent weakness, but they are nearly always strongly influenced by aberrant nerve impulses.

Nervous tension and stress are major players in the formation and continuance of strictures. Because of these mechanical blockages, elimination is often poor when nervous strain and emotional upset are present. Therefore, it is of primary importance that stricture conditions be treated with consideration of the aberrant nerve impulses due to both physical and emotional causes. Once the nervous pathways associated with strictures are formed, I doubt it's possible for them to be completely eliminated. Nerve impulses will always tend to follow well-established routes. But it is possible to make both physical and mental corrections so that bowel strictures can become manageable.

FLATULENCE

Many things can cause flatulence (bowel gas). Certain chemical processes in the colon produce various gases as byproducts of normal bowel function. Some, such as carbon dioxide, are odorless, while others, such as hydrogen sulfide, are very odorous. Bowel gas is of little consequence in a healthy colon. This isn't true, however, in a diseased or dysfunctional colon. Excessive bowel gas is an indication of bowel disturbance and can be very serious in its consequences. For example, when there is a bowel stricture or fecal obstruction as in constipation, the gaseous products may become trapped. Trapped bowel gases can result in extreme pressure, which can manifest as distention and/or pain. When there are diverticula or ballooning in the bowel, trapped waste accumulates. These conditions often cause putrefactive fermentation, which results in considerable gas, discomfort, and reabsorption of toxins into the body, followed by autointoxication.

Once a bowel has diverticula, it will never be entirely free of gas. Because diverticula are so very common, there are few people who can say they have no bowel gas whatsoever. Getting the gas out completely is almost an impossibility, not only because of the prevalence of diverticular disease, but because diet and lifestyle seldom can be modified to the extent necessary to accomplish this task. I do think, however, that with proper attention to diet, gas can be reduced so that it will cause little disturbance, distress, or social embarrassment.

Reducing gas in the bowel nearly always means making a change in the diet. If you suffer from gas problems, find out whether any specific foods are a cause. Eliminate these foods from your diet, or consume them in limited quantities along with foods that are not gas-producing.

Some foods can cause a lot of gas in some people and little or none in others. Consuming too much starch and protein tends to cause a lot of gas. The proteins usually consumed by persons in the United States include red meat, fish, fowl, and dairy products. Although I feel that these animal proteins are not necessarily troublesome if consumed in moderate amounts, they may present serious gas problems for some persons. This is especially true when, for various reasons, protein digestion is incomplete.

When undigested proteins find their way into the colon, they provide nourishment for undesirable bacteria, helping them to multiply. These undesirable bacteria are responsible for the breakdown of organic compounds by way of a putrefactive process. This process is undesirable specifically because the bacteria produce metabolic wastes that are toxic, disease-producing, and gas-producing. Some of the waste materials they produce are injurious to bodily tissues. These organisms were not intended to inhabit the human bowel in significant numbers. Bacteria that are beneficial and, indeed, necessary for good health cannot live in a bowel that is dirty, gaseous, toxic, constipated, and overrun with organisms of the unfriendly sort.

Beans and other legumes are roughly half protein and half starch. They tend to cause a lot of gas because of certain indigestible sugars in the starch. These sugars (stachyose, verbascose, and raffinose) arrive intact in the lower intestine, where the bacteria digest them, releasing the byproducts of carbon dioxide, hydrogen, and sometimes methane. Other foods that are naturally gas-forming include the sulfur foods such as broccoli, cabbage, and onions. The sulfur foods seem to cause more gas problems when cooked than when raw. If it is necessary to cook sulfur vegetables, cook them in covered, stainless-steel waterless cookware over very low heat only until they are tender yet firm, not soggy.

I have found that consuming nuts, especially peanuts, and too much roughage can also cause a lot of gas. Dried fruit eaten directly from the bag can cause gas problems. Dried fruit can be rehydrated by being boiled and soaked overnight. (For complete directions, see Appendix A.) The next morning, the fruit will approximate fresh fruit and not cause gas problems.

Although we are told that eating raw foods is desirable, we are not often told that doing so without having gas problems requires a healthy bowel with a fairly rapid transit time. Although raw foods do promote a more rapid bowel transit time, persons with a chronically sluggish colon may not be wise to consume them in great quantities. Raw foods, as well as live foods (foods that have not had their enzymes destroyed by the heat of cooking), can produce a lot of gas in a sluggish, slow-moving bowel. More raw foods can be consumed as bowel function improves and should be slowly introduced over a period of time to allow the body to make adjustments.

To eliminate extreme gas conditions, we should first consider the foods we eat. When spoiled food is eaten, it continues to spoil in the small intestine and then in the large intestine. This process of putrefaction produces gas. Animal proteins—especially ground-up meats such as those found in hamburgers, hot dogs, sausages, and some cold cuts—putrefy easily in the warmth of the digestive tract. This is because each cell in meat has a sac of enzymes called lysozymes whose purpose is to chemically break down and digest the cell. When meat is ground, the sac ruptures and the enzymes flood the cell, acting as a kind of built-in self-destruct apparatus. This is why ground meat always spoils quicker than meat that is left intact. So, when you consume ground meat, you have a head start on the putrefaction process.

Another reason meat, fish, and poultry can cause gas in some persons is that these foods are deficient in fiber and thus not moved along well by peristalsis, resulting in increased transit time. When transit time is slowed, foods have more time to putrefy, a process accelerated by the 98.6°F (Fahrenheit) temperature of the body. It is this break-down (putrefaction) process that results in gas. Fairly rapid transit time and no worries about gas are as desirable for the bowel as they are for public transportation. Therefore, if animal proteins are eaten, a sufficient quantity of high-fiber foods must be consumed along with them to help decrease transit time and rid the colon of waste products before putrefaction can become a gas-producing problem. Although this is especially true of animal proteins, it also holds true for vegetable proteins and, to a lesser degree, all foods.

We should also be aware of the role of liquids. Drinking a quantity of liquids with meals can cause gas. On the other hand, soup, broth, juice, or water taken between meals can cut down on the amount of bowel gas. Be aware of the air you swallow, too. Many people gulp air when they eat, especially when they eat too fast. Whipped foods contain a lot of air and can be the cause of gas troubles. Some medications, both prescription and over-the-counter, can interfere with bowel activity. Some are stimulants, and laxatives must be included in this category. Antihistamines, antibiotics, and sulfa drugs are great contributors to gastrointestinal problems, including gas, as they destroy the friendly bacteria in the intestine. Drug residues can settle in the tissues of the bowel wall and continue to cause problems.

Bowel gas can be a problem for persons who lack sufficient digestive enzymes to properly process food into a state in which it can be absorbed. As we age, the body's production of enzymes in the saliva, hydrochloric acid in the stomach, and additional digestive enzymes from the pancreas is reduced. Certain diseases, blockages, and dysfunctional states may also diminish the availability of these enzymes and acids. In these cases, ingested foods will proceed through the small intestine to the lower bowel along with a large quantity of partially digested food. This partially digested food will then putrefy and produce gas. It may be helpful in this case to take, with meals, a digestive-enzyme supplement or, in some cases, a hydrochloric-acid supplement.

Persons who suffer from bowel gas will find that mint tea or an extract of mint is a great gas-driver. Wild yam extract is also wonderful. For an irritated bowel, I recommend flaxseed tea. (For a recipe, see page 120.) Flaxseed tea with a teaspoon of liquid chlorophyll assists in relieving the irritated conditions in the bowel that can produce a lot of gas and disturbance. Rice and barley gruel also help with gas disturbances, as do apples, which are very high in organic sodium and potassium, and feed the bowel wall with these necessary minerals. A deficiency of these minerals causes the bowel wall to weaken, which results in the intestinal contents not being acted upon or propelled along with the proper intensity. This weakening may even help produce diverticula. Also, sluggishness increases transit time, allowing more gas-producing fermentation to occur. As mentioned, digestive aids, pancreatic enzymes, hydrochloric-acid tablets, and friendly-bacteria supplements all help the bowel to eliminate gas. Don't forget that avoiding gas-producing foods and foods that destroy friendly bacteria also help.

Friendly Bacteria

Bulgaria has traditionally had more people living past one hundred years of age per capita than any other country in the world. The Bulgarians claim this is because their diet includes a fair amount of clabbered milk, which contains the *Lactobacillus bulgaricus* bacteria. Anyone with a bowel problem should take a course of lactobacillus culture for at least one month three times a year.

One thing I learned from Dr. John Harvey Kellogg is that we have "friendly" bacteria in the bowel. These friendly bacteria keep the bowel clean and hold the "unfriendly" bacteria in check. This helps to create a balance that minimizes putrefaction and fermentation, the producers of excess gas and bad odors. Dr. Kellogg taught that the correct bacterial balance for a healthy bowel is about 85-percent friendly lactobacillus bacteria and 15-percent unfriendly, gas-producing *Bacillus coli.*

I wanted to find out about the intestinal flora—the various bacteria, both friendly and unfriendly, that populate the bowel—of my patients. I sent fecal samples from five hundred patients to a medical laboratory to find out the relative amounts of friendly and unfriendly bacteria. The lab results averaged 85-percent unfriendly bacteria and 15-percent friendly bacteria, just the opposite of what they should have been! This taught me that the bowels of most people are not what they should be from the standpoint of having a healthy balance of intestinal flora. Is it any wonder that we have so much trouble with bowel gas?

We should be aware that animal protein (meat) can reduce the numbers of friendly bacteria in the bowel. When consumed in excess, animal protein feeds and favors the multiplication of unfriendly bacteria at the expense of friendly bacteria—especially in the presence of a lazy colon. The caffeine in coffee and chocolate also reduces the number of friendly bacteria. It may surprise some readers that nearly all cooked foods, especially overcooked foods, are inadequate for feeding friendly intestinal bacteria, whereas raw foods encourage the establishment and maintenance of balanced intestinal flora. A more proper floral balance in the bowel can be restored by reducing the intake of cooked foods and by supplementing the diet with friendly bacterial cultures. Various cultures of friendly bacteria are available in supplement form. (See "Probiotic Supplementation" on page 137.)

Although these dietary suggestions are essential for gas elimination, reducing bowel gas has been one of the most difficult things to accomplish through diet. When we begin changing our diet and start eating natural high-fiber foods that have not been manhandled, we find that we often have more of a gas condition than we had before. Consuming these foods is like stirring up a dirty basement—as we sweep the floor clean, a lot of dust gets in the air. Roughage is the broom that moves the waste out of distentions and diverticula, temporarily creating additional gas. This gas will decrease as the bowel becomes cleaner and proper function is restored.

In taking care of people who had begun to adopt a better diet, I noticed an unusual circumstance. Those who were suffering with a lot of bowel gas could resort to the worst possible diet, returning to their old habits, and their gas problems would abate. When we put them back on the high-fiber diet, they again had gas to contend with.

However, they said they were passing the gas more easily and their stools had become softer. They no longer had to force bowel movements. Their feces moved through the bowel more easily, and their constipation was gone. Even though the gas problem persisted for a while, it continued to gradually lessen until it was minimal and not bothersome.

Whenever there is gas and it cannot be taken care of through an ordinary food routine or ordinary treatments, I know it is a very serious problem indeed. I believe that long before serious gas symptoms appear in the body, there are long-standing preconditions in the bowel, and we should be able to see how to take care of these things before symptoms appear.

ULCERATION

Ulceration of the bowel occurs due to irritation, abrasion, infection, and concentrated toxins settling in or on sensitive tissues. Ulcerations can be the result of improper diet, mental distress, inharmonious living, radiation burns, aberrant nerve impulses associated with spinal misalignment, cancer, and opportunistic infections. Ulcers can also be secondary to other digestive disorders.

Ulceration results in open sores, bleeding, and pain, as is common with gastric and duodenal ulcers. The sigmoid and rectum in the lower bowel are the sites of most of these troubles, although the upper gastrointestinal tract is also prone to ulcerations. The mouth, esophagus, and, of course, the stomach and duodenum are common sites as well.

Ulcerations should be treated with the same concern as other bowel disorders. Finding and removing the cause is always the best thing to do. Ulcerations secondary to other health problems should be dealt with accordingly. Diet and lifestyle should be considered in any therapy or management program.

BOWEL SPASM

Bowel spasm, as seen in Figure 3.4, is a chronic tightening of the muscle fibers due to hyperactivity of the nerve impulses controlling muscle action. A rather common condition, it frequently manifests as constipation alternating with diarrhea. When present, bowel spasm is usually found in the descending, sigmoid, or ascending portions of the colon and is somewhat more rare in the transverse segment. Bowel spasm is often associated with colitis and diverticulitis. When any muscle is overworked, irritated, and tense, it will go into spasm.

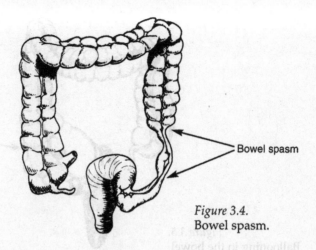

Bowel spasm

Figure 3.4.
Bowel spasm.

Over time, muscle spasm in an area of the colon often leads to a ballooned condition immediately preceding the spastic area. (See Figure 3.5.) This is due to pressure and a backup of feces created by the restriction of the spasm. It's easy in this instance to see how one colon problem can lead to additional problems until the entire digestive tract is influenced.

It is interesting to note that people who suffer with spasms in the colon, which may or may not be associated with colitis, nearly always have psychological problems or are under a great deal of stress. Worries, fears, anxieties, grief, and similar problems often cause aberrant nerve impulses to flow in the nervous system. The digestive tract is always the recipient of these impulses. There is a little sign posted in a number of diners across the land that reads, "You don't get ulcers from what you eat; you get them from what's eating you." There's more truth to that statement than is generally thought. Although diet certainly plays an important role in all digestive conditions, persons with spasms, irritable bowel syndrome, and colitis must also seek counseling for help in dealing with their inward feelings and stressful situations before their colon problems can be effectively addressed.

Sometimes, when there is no mental or stressful counterpart to a spasm condition, a spinal misalignment may be the cause of the problem. A chiropractor or physical therapist may be able to help with this.

ADHESIONS
Adhesions of the colon are caused by inflammation and irritation of the bowel wall. Inflammation and irritation can cause the mucous

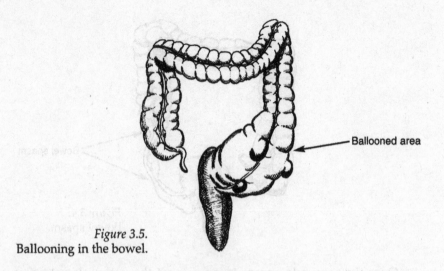

Figure 3.5.
Ballooning in the bowel.

membrane of the bowel to break down to such an extent that a raw, irritated, exposed surface develops. If there is more than one surface area like this and they are close to one another, they can stick together due to gluelike substances that are secreted from the open tissues. Although this sticking process is part of normal wound healing, it can cause the joining of tissues that should not be joined. Such undesirable adhesions sometimes occur following surgical procedures. Adhesions can be a serious condition that sometimes requires delicate surgery.

BOWEL PARASITES

Although not strictly a bowel disorder, parasites thrive in an unhealthy, unclean intestine. When the bowel contains partially digested proteins, it can harbor an amazing variety of harmful bacteria and parasites.

Parasites are the number-one health enemy in the world. A nationwide survey reported by the *Chicago Tribune* utilized 414,820 samples of feces examined at 570 public and private laboratories in all fifty states and revealed that 1 of every 6 persons studied had one or more parasites. The parasites ranged from microscopic organisms to fifteen-foot tapeworms.

It is estimated that 200,000,000 people are infected with these intestinal invaders. In fact, intestinal worms of various types outrank cancer as mankind's deadliest enemy worldwide. Although not a major problem in the United States, the people in this country are not immune to worms, and the number of cases of worm infestation has been increasing in recent years. In supervising the Ultimate Tissue Cleansing Program, I have seen a variety of worms passed by quite a few people. Often, these people were greatly surprised at finding out they had harbored parasites.

Intestinal parasites can enter the body in several ways. By far the most common means is through food or water contaminated with the parasite. Food or water may also contain the eggs or larvae of parasites. Some parasites, as well as their eggs and larvae, may not be affected by the harsh hydrochloric acid of the stomach or the juices of the intestine, and so are able to survive the journey to the intestinal region that is most favorable to their development.

A common example of parasites that survive the acids and enzymes of the upper digestive tract is *Enterobius vennicularis*, also known as pinworms. Pinworm infestation, called enterobiasis, is common among children, even in the United States. It is probably safe to say that nearly every child will contract pinworms at some time and perhaps several times. The worms are not particularly harmful, but produce an annoying rectal itch when they exit the anus at night to lay their tiny eggs around the orifice, covering the eggs with an irritating sticky substance that causes the itch. When the anal area is scratched in response to the itch, eggs are picked up on the fingers. If the fingers are brought into contact with the mouth, as small children tend to do, the eggs are ingested and survive the rigors of the upper digestive tract to infect the lower bowel once again. This cycle of reinfection can be broken only by preventing the fingers from coming near the mouth. When this is done, the infection usually dies out after a few days. Although pinworms are very common and not a serious threat to health, other worm infestations, such as trichinosis, can be very serious. No worm infestation should be taken lightly.

It is more common to harbor parasites when the intestinal flora are unbalanced and the digestive tract, especially the colon, is dirty and pocketed. Under these conditions, the colon becomes a breeding ground for parasites, much the same as a garbage dump is a perfect breeding ground for rats. All life tends to migrate to a place where the conditions are most favorable for its continued development. Worms and other intestinal parasites are no exception. This is yet another reason to keep the diet and the bowel as clean as possible.

The symptoms of parasitic infection include abdominal pain, nausea, vomiting, and chronic diarrhea. Parasitic infections, however, are often misdiagnosed. A good way to deter or eradicate parasites is to consume garlic or the herb black walnut.

PROLAPSUS

Prolapsus refers to the sinking or falling down of a body part. Prolapse of the colon, shown in Figure 3.6, is a very common occurrence. The portion of the colon most likely to prolapse is the transverse colon, the section that travels across the upper abdomen. When the transverse colon prolapses, it places pressure upon the abdominal contents below it, and pulls or draws on the organs above it. Before we consider the various complications that can arise from prolapse of the colon, let's see what causes it to sag in the first place.

Prolapsus is often associated with chemical (nutritional) imbalances in the body and also with constipation. These two things, combined with the more or less constant force of gravity acting upon the body, cause the contents of this section of the abdomen to sag. The transverse colon has the softest tissue in the body, and it is the only structure that extends horizontally across the upper abdomen from one side of the body to the other. If it were hard, like bone, it could not drop from gravity. Because it is soft, however, it is more easily affected by gravitational force.

The intestines are supported by ligaments and a tough, fatty covering called the greater omentum. The greater omentum cushions the bowel from excessive trauma and vibration, and keeps it from moving about, but it is primarily the ligamentous tissues that keep the higher part of the bowel from falling down and putting pressure on the lower abdominal organs. Ligaments, like any other bodily tissue, have certain nutritional requirements to remain in optimum health. Although exercise should not be forgotten, tissues of any type are best

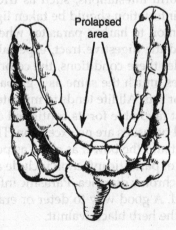

Prolapsed
area

Figure 3.6.
Prolapse of the colon.

maintained when they are fed the minerals and other nutrients necessary for their repair and regeneration. When the ligaments holding the bowel are in good repair, the bowel will not sag.

Minerals are the most important structural elements in the body. Although the majority of people think of vitamins and enzymes as being the most important nutrients required by humans, it is minerals that constitute the essential components of the structure of tissues. Vitamins and enzymes facilitate chemical reactions and processes in the body, but do not constitute the structure of tissues. Minerals, on the other hand, are the basic components of tissues. Although your automobile certainly needs gasoline and oil in order to function, its composition and strength are largely due to the steel and other structural materials. When there is a structural failure, you need to replace a part, not just add fuel and oil. In like manner, weak ligaments need the mineral manganese for repair and regeneration. When the ligaments lack manganese, they become weak and can no longer resist the force of gravity. Thus, they become stretched, which results in a sagging of the organs they are designed to support.

Recently, the FDA determined that 40 percent of the country's population suffers from a lack of calcium. Calcium is especially needed for the repair and maintenance of bones and for proper muscle function. This is one example of a mineral that finally has come to the attention of health authorities in a dramatic way because osteoporosis (calcium-depleted bones) in postmenopausal women has nearly reached epidemic proportions in the United States. It has been found that affected women did not receive enough calcium during their child-bearing years. Often these women develop what is known as a dowager's hump, an extreme curvature of the thoracic spine, due to vertebral compression of the calcium-deficient bones. The resulting stooped posture puts pressure on the abdominal contents, helping to force the colon into a prolapsed condition.

Another problem that can contribute to prolapse of the colon is constipation. When the intestinal contents back up, from whatever cause, fecal material becomes dry and impacted. Long-term improper bowel care results in a thick buildup of mucus on the colon wall. The combination of fecal material and mucus causes the transverse colon to become very heavy with material that should move on. The weight of this material, combined with poor nutrition to the muscles and ligaments plus the force of gravity, results in prolapsus.

Fatigue contributes to prolapsus as well. I have often said that fatigue is present at the beginning of every disease. When we are tired, gravity has its most profound effects on us. Muscle tone is lost, so the internal organs are more easily pulled downward. When fatigue takes its toll, our shoulders begin to droop. Abnormal sideways curvature of the spine may develop, and the normal curvatures of the spine may become accentuated.

When prolapse of the colon occurs, pressure is exerted on the abdominal organs below. The constant pressure on these tissues not only imposes an increased load on their suspensory ligaments, but decreases the supply of blood and lymph to the areas where the pressure is applied. This can result in abnormal growths, toxic-waste buildup, and stretching, as well as compression of tissues, even displacements. As the colon sags, it pulls down the structures above it, which can result in a fishhook shaping of the stomach with pooling of stomach acid in the lowest part of that organ. Prolapse of the uterus and tipping of the uterus, as well as bladder, vaginal, uterine, and ovarian tumors are often associated with a prolapsed colon.

We sometimes find that in women, there is pressure on the fallopian tubes and the ovaries. Occasionally, eggs released from the ovaries cannot pass into the uterus properly, which can cause sterility. We also find that women have more cysts on the ovaries than on any other organ in the body. Women undergo hysterectomies more than any other operation, and I believe this is because a good deal of pressure is exerted against the tubes, pressure that does not allow the proper circulation of blood or the removal of toxic material from the uterus.

In men, pressure on the prostate gland can result in prostate congestion or dysfunction. The urethra, through which the urine flows from the bladder, passes through the center of the prostate gland. When there is enough pressure on the prostate gland, urination is difficult. Urine, a liquid that can be absorbed back into the body, will be retained. Some health professionals believe that urine retention and its effects on blood chemistry may be linked to the beginning of arthritis and joint troubles, especially as we grow older. Circulating toxic materials tend to settle in the areas of the body farthest from the heart because the circulation is poorest there. The toxins often affect the joints in the arms, legs, feet, and hands. Arthritics usually complain of pain and stiffness in the extremities.

We find that prostate-gland and bladder troubles, and uterine and ovarian disturbances may all be associated with prolapsus. We know, too, that many gastrointestinal specialists and other doctors make their living treating hemorrhoids and other anal, rectal, and bowel problems caused mainly by pressure from the transverse colon. So pervasive is prolapse of the transverse colon that it is rare these days to see an adult without some evidence of this condition.

The pressure of prolapsus can be relieved by regular use of a slant board, a piece of equipment normally found in gyms but also available as a portable or home unit. (See "Exercise" on page 140.) With the aid of this board, you can lie supine with your legs elevated and head down, a position the reverse of normal that allows gravitational force to relieve the prolapsus. Spending a few minutes each day lying on a slant board helps to return prolapsed abdominal organs to their original positions and combats fatigue.

COLON CANCER

The second leading cause of death in the United States is cancer, and every year 100,000 Americans lose their lives to colon cancer. Recently, the American Cancer Society issued a statement saying, "Evidence in recent years suggests that most bowel cancer is caused by environmental agents. Some scientists believe that a diet high in beef and/or low in fiber is the cause." In fact, literature from the American Cancer Society now extols the benefits of fresh fruits and vegetables, especially the cruciform vegetables such as broccoli, Brussels sprouts, and cabbage, uncooked or lightly steamed. In the recent past, doctors and scientists who thought diet plays a role in cancer were considered to be food faddists or quacks. The faddists included Denis P. Burkitt, M.D., the famous English surgeon who claimed in as early as 1972 that diet plays a role in many diseases including cancer.

Now that it has become more or less common knowledge that diet plays a vital role in cancer prevention, it is prudent to say that bowel cleansing also has its place in preventing cancer as well as other diseases. People can get into a lot of trouble making claims about diseases, especially cancer. Cancer is a sensitive and explosive issue, not only because it is a multibillion-dollar industry, but also because the disease carries a lot of emotional freight as well. We dare not say that bowel cleansing helps prevent cancer, but anyone can see that cleanliness and restoration of proper function go a long way toward building resistance to disease of any kind.

IN CONCLUSION

I do not wish to give the impression that I have become one-sided in my emphasis upon a healthy, clean intestinal tract, but the evidence I've seen over a long period of time indicates people do not realize that toxic accumulation is at the root of most of our diseases today. Furthermore, people do not regard poor health to be as serious a problem as they should. They place their health problems secondary to all their other problems—real and imagined—but the health of an individual or a nation should always be the first concern. Without health, there is little that you can truly enjoy.

Never before have people lived in such a toxic environment. Our air, water, food, soil, clothing, and everything we touch has the potential of being toxic to our system, as environmental pollutants gain entry to the body by various routes. When we have toxic substances in our colon seeping into our bodily tissues, it's like we have a time-released poison in our bowel. The poison works slowly, imperceptibly wearing down the vitality, resistance, and health of our bodily tissues and organs. It's as though we have our own personal toxic-waste site that we carry around with us. When the colon is toxic, it continually serves up microdoses of poison to the blood.

The need to detoxify and cleanse the body has never been greater than right now. People are more toxic-ridden today than ever in known history. The widespread existence of toxic substances and the levels at which they are found are becoming a nightmare as illness continues to take its toll. Nearly all the patients I see have some kind of bowel disorder associated with toxicity, even if they are unaware of it.

Restoring balance, peace, and harmony is the physician's job. That is the task he has chosen. However, it cannot be done effectively or lastingly in a body that is breaking down due to an accumulation of toxic materials. When we cleanse and remove the toxic debris; feed the body good, healthy, vital foods; and stop poisoning ourselves, the body will respond with healing and reversal of the disease processes.

The road to health begins with an understanding of and commitment to cleansing and detoxifying the body and restoring balance, peace, and harmony. Too few people in our culture experience the benefits of proper bowel function. Too few people live in a manner that enables them to maintain the natural balance of the body. If we are going to live unnaturally, we would be wise to learn how to counteract some of the maladies we create in our personal environment.

Chapter 4

The Neural-Arc Reflex

This chapter is very special to me. It is my story. It is the result of my many years of work and experience with thousands of people at my sanitariums, as well as with my own bowel problems.

At age seventy-six, I experienced problems with my left hip and leg. I went to five or six chiropractors in the hope that they could help me. Even though their techniques and therapies were masterful, I received only the most temporary relief. It shortly became obvious that my problem did not lend itself to joint manipulation or chiropractic spinal adjustment alone. I needed something additional. I visited my family physician to see what he could do, but this approach wasn't helpful either. After giving much careful thought to the situation, I decided to take the matter into my own hands, remaining ever mindful of the dictum, "The person who treats himself has a fool for a patient and an idiot for a doctor." Nevertheless, for better or for worse, I thought it was time to see if I could do for myself what others had failed to do. I began by having a complete barium study done of my lower intestinal tract.

During a lower gastrointestinal (GI) study, the colon is filled with liquid barium via the rectum, and, under mild pressure, the barium goes into any diverticula that may exist. The barium shows up white on the X-rays, providing a crisp, clear outline of the bowel wall and diverticula, as well as any other irregularities.

It became clearly and instantly evident that I had a fairly large diverticulum in my colon. Confirming this with an X-ray, I began in earnest to take steps to detoxify my colon by making improvements

81

in my diet, consuming foods high in fiber, and taking regular supplements of bran and psyllium seed. I also added more exercise to my personal health regimen. As my bowel movements became more regular and copious over a period of two weeks, my hip and leg troubles left me.

The doctors I had seen were very good clinicians, but they all had failed to make the connection between my hip and leg symptoms and my bowel. Even though I have been teaching people about proper diet, bowel care, and exercise nearly all of my adult life, I was greatly impressed by my personal experience with the relationship between diverticula in specific locations and problems in specific parts of the body. While my studies and observations of patients over many years had led me to accept this concept intellectually, nothing was as convincing as personally experiencing the phenomenon.

Not too many years ago, I gave a name to this phenomenon of certain areas of the bowel being linked to certain parts of the body. I called the phenomenon the neural-arc reflex, a name based on the physiological phenomenon of involuntary response to a stimulus. (For the story of how I made "My Greatest Discovery," see below.)

My Greatest Discovery

In the days when doctors still made house calls, when I was just breaking into the healing arts, Dr. Glen Sipes asked me to accompany him on an emergency house call to Oakland, California. We arrived to find a young man in his thirties in bed with a high fever, his skin as red as a beet and all his joints filled with great pain. Dr. Sipes percussed (tapped) the man's abdomen over the bowel, listening carefully. He asked the patient, "Did you have a bowel movement today?"

The patient answered, "No."

"Did you have a bowel movement yesterday?" Dr. Sipes asked.

"No," the young man said.

"When did you have your last bowel movement?" the doctor asked.

"I don't remember."

Dr. Sipes then asked the patient's mother to prepare an enema, but the woman didn't know what an enema was. Dr. Sipes therefore went out into the yard, cut a piece of reed with his pocket knife, and hollowed the reed out with a piece of baling wire. Back in the house, he had the patient's mother heat some water. He then inserted one end of the hollow reed into the man's anus and blew mouthfuls of warm water into the rectum. After repeated enemas, the patient's fever went down, his skin color returned to normal, and his pain disappeared. This all took place in less than an hour.

I could hardly believe that such great relief could come to a person just from taking care of the bowel. This made a believer out of me! I had seen it with my own eyes.

A while later, I spent some time with Dr. Max Gerson at his sanitarium in New Jersey. Dr. Gerson was a medical doctor who used enemas to clean his patients' bowels. He wrote a book entitled *Fifty Cancer Patients Cured*. Watching Dr. Gerson confirmed my faith in bowel cleansing, but as yet I wasn't sure why the technique worked.

When I read the works of Sir W. Arbuthnot Lane, physician to the British Royal Family, I saw that his surgeries to cut out diseased parts of the colon sometimes resulted in complete relief of diseases elsewhere in the body such as arthritis, asthma, and toxic thyroid. I thought, "There has to be a connection between the condition of the bowel and the other parts of the body, but what is it?" I felt like a detective on the track of some great mystery.

During all this time, a period of many years, I was familiar with Hering's Law of Cure. Dr. Constantine Hering, a European homeopath, had come to this country and established a homeopathic college in Philadelphia. He had claimed, "All cure starts from within out, from the head down, and in the reverse order as the symptoms appeared." This law is a "sleeper." It has never been properly used. Dr. Hering knew what he was talking about, but I don't think other homeopaths knew what he meant. I didn't see the connection to the bowel at first either. I thought Dr. Hering's law had to do with toxemia and its treatment by fasting, as taught by John Tilden, M.D., in his book *Toxemia Explained*. I hadn't quite caught on yet.

During this time, in the 1940s, I had patients with pain in a specific part of their bowel who also had cancer or another serious condition in some other part of their body. Some of the patients, through fasting, a specialized diet, or other cleansing work, reported complete remission of their degenerative condition. I was getting wonderful results with patients, teaching them how to work for a healing crisis. A healing crisis is the crisis point during which the body works the hardest to rid itself of mucus and catarrh. Old symptoms reappear and resolve. The bowel elimination is often unbelievable. A healing crisis usually lasts from three to seven days and always brings a wonderful reversal of some chronic condition. And, the bowel is always involved the crisis.

I remembered movie star Rudolph Valentino, who died after a series of surgeries for bowel problems. From that time on, I watched for the obituaries of well-known entertainers and politicians, and was surprised at how many died from complications involving one or more of the elimination channels. At the same time, I was learning that when the bowel is underactive, the other elimination channels—the skin, kidneys, lymphatic system, and lungs—are overtaxed. So many things point back to the bowel when something is wrong in the body and during a healing crisis. I wondered, "What is the key to this thing?" I was convinced by then that there is a reflex relationship between conditions in the bowel and conditions in the other organs, glands, and tissues of the body.

I learned that tons of laxatives were being sold every year because constipation and other causes of bowel underactivity are so widespread. About 80 percent of the people who visit a doctor have a chronic disease. Was there a connection?

Possibly due to overwork, I was suffering my own bowel problems and began to take what were called colema treatments from Kay Shaffer, a nurse who was a student of Dr. V.E. Irons. The colemas helped me, and I began using them in my own bowel work, even developing the Ultimate Tissue Cleansing Program. My knowledge and understanding of the bowel was growing, and I was getting better results with my patients.

To learn more about the bowel reflex, which I named the neural-arc reflex, I began to study embryology. I learned that by the second week of formation, the embryo takes the shape of the primitive "gut tube," and its nervous system begins to form. This means that the bowel tissue and nerve tissue are very intimately related. (See Figure 4.1 on page 91.) By the fourth week, buds such as the lung bud and liver bud begin to bulge out from the gut and nerve tissue. By the sixth week, most of the organ buds begin to form. These organ buds, I suddenly noticed, are covered with a membrane made up of the same tissue that formed the bowel and nerve tissue in the earlier embryo. That was when I realized that the tissue of the primitive gut surrounds each organ with a membrane.

All of a sudden it came to me. This is how the genetic weaknesses of the mother and father are passed down to the children—through the gut and nerve tissue that becomes the membrane covering the organs. Where the bowel has an inherent weakness, the organ that developed from that area of the bowel also has an inherent weakness. *This is the key to the neural-arc syndrome.* I could now see how certain areas of the bowel were reflexly related to specific organs. Any genetic weakness in the bowel could affect the performance of the organ associated with that part of the bowel. Toxicity or nutrient depletion in one would affect the other. This makes that part of the bowel and that organ more subject to breakdown and consequently to diseases.

I refer to genetically weak tissue as an "inherent weakness," and most of my students and patients understand that by an inherently weak organ I mean an organ that is more vulnerable to nutrient depletion and toxic encumbrances than "normal" organs. An inherently weak organ is more subject to breakdown and disease. We all have these inherent weaknesses from birth, and they will be with us for a lifetime. *As it is in the embryo, so it will be all through life.*

Autointoxication due to underactive elimination channels soon brings on enervation and fatigue. This is what Dr. Tilden taught. The beginning of all disease is toxemia and enervation. I was able to prove what Dr. Tilden taught. His theories were right, but he didn't know why. I know why. I put it all together and saw the whole picture.

We start out in life with our parents' various inherent weaknesses. Our health depends a good deal on what our parents passed on to us. We all begin life with a few things against us, a few inherently weak areas in the bowel. Normally, if an adverse condition develops in an inherently weak part of the bowel, it will reflex to some other part of the body, causing a problem possibly very remote from the source of the trouble. Because of the lack of pain nerves in the bowel, the patient doesn't complain about the bowel, and the doctor has no reason to suspect that the problem is in the bowel. So, the doctor treats the sinuses, or the shoulder, or the pancreas, while the source of the problem remains unchanged. You can see from what I have described that wherever the weakness was in the gut directly reflexes to the organ that grew out of the gut in that place. To take care of inherent weaknesses, we must take care of the whole person! But, always the bowel first. If we take good care of the bowel, we can make the most of it and have better health as a result.

When I understood this, Hering's Law of Cure came alive to me! "All cure starts from within out [from the bowel reflexing to other parts of the body], from the head down [from the organ-control centers in the brain influencing the organs they are connected to], and in the reverse order as the symptoms appeared [with the reversal being due to a healing crisis and the elimination of any toxic material associated with both the bowel and the organs involved in the disease condition]."

I could see it all: The bowel is king. And if we take care of the king, he will take care of his kingdom—our body. This is why it is so important to take care of the bowel—to keep it clean and well-nourished. If we take care of our living habits, nutrition, and thinking, we will take care of any inherent weaknesses in the bowel and any organs that are reflexly affected. We must take care of inherent weaknesses. Inherent strengths will take care of themselves.

While bowel cleansing is not a cure-all, there is no one I have ever treated who didn't feel better when new tissue replaced the old. That is why I feel this is "my greatest discovery." I have often wondered why I get such good results with my patients. Since my discovery, I have realized it is because I always take care of the bowel first. I have many testimonials from patients who have taken my counsel on nutrition and elimination, and have experienced better health. For each of those testimonials, I have hundreds of additional patients who are thankful for a new start in life. It isn't necessary for everyone to take colemas to achieve wonderful results. But nature is slow, and colemas quicken the work of healing and tissue removal. Bowel cleansing, after all, is a natural healing art, not a treatment art.

These involuntary responses, or reflexes, are similar to such occurrences as a knee jerk when the area below the knee is struck with a doctor's reflex hammer. The neural-arc reflex occurs when a portion of the bowel is irritated by the toxins associated with static, putrefactive debris, and aberrant nerve impulses are transmitted, via nervous pathways, to a remote area. These impulses cause symptoms to occur reflexly in the remote area. In other words, there is a relationship between certain organs, glands, and tissues, and certain parts of the bowel. There was a relationship between the dirty bowel pocket I saw on my X-ray and the symptoms I was experiencing in my hip and leg. Treating the hip and leg with various therapies did nothing to get at the root cause of the problem. As long as the colon condition remained untreated, the symptoms persisted. The neural-arc reflex is the perfect example of why the bowel is the king of the elimination channels.

Consider how the body's neurological function is similar to the workings of a modern pipe organ. A modern pipe organ can be played from a remote console, with the pipe-work producing the sound possibly being quite far removed from the console. This is made possible by a complex array of electrical connections that serve to link the controls at the console with the hundreds, or perhaps thousands, of pipes residing in the distant chamber. Consider, too, that the great composer Wolfgang Amadeus Mozart called the pipe organ the "king of instruments" because it is the largest and most complex musical instrument ever made and because it is so versatile that it can mimic quite a number of different instruments. Bowel problems can cause symptoms that mimic a multitude of diseases, and doctors are quite familiar with complaints of pain in one area that are caused by a problem in another area. Physicians call this referred pain.

Referred pain is actually a rather common occurrence. Pain or any symptom experienced in one part of the body but stemming from a condition in a different location can present a diagnostic challenge for an examining physician. This situation can be quite puzzling to the patient as well. A common example of referred pain is the pain that is sometimes experienced in the right shoulder but stems from a gall-bladder attack. Another common example of referred pain is the pain that is experienced in the left arm but stems from a heart condition. No pathology exists in the shoulder or arm itself. In cases of referred pain, it would be ineffectual in the least and perhaps even dangerous to treat the pain site while leaving the cause of the problem unattended.

Referred pain demonstrates how, just as in a pipe organ, the connections of the body are manifold and complex. By comparison, however, the body's connections make the musical instrument seem elementary. The real "king of instruments" is the human body. The digestive tract is the great console of the body. It can be the creator of harmony or disharmony. Disharmony occurring in the digestive tract has its sounding board in areas of the body removed from the gut. The nervous system, via countless pathways, connects the walls of the digestive tract to every corner of the body. Because of this neurological and anatomical fact, the bowel reigns supreme.

The bowel is the king of the five main organs of elimination. It is the hub of the digestive system. The bowel is one of the largest structures in the body, taking up more room than any other internal structure. Please remember that the digestive tract actually begins with the mouth and extends to the anus. Thus it includes the throat, esophagus, stomach, small intestine, and large intestine. The large intestine, as already noted, is often referred to as the lower bowel or colon, and includes the ascending colon with its appendix and the transverse colon with its two curvatures, or flexures. Then there is the descending colon, which is immediately followed by the rectum and the anus. Each section of the intestinal tract has a particular function that contributes to the smooth operation of the entire digestive mechanism. All in all, the total length of this intestinal plumbing approaches thirty feet!

GETTING TO THE ROOT OF THE PROBLEM

Some years ago, there was a popular television miniseries called *Roots*. It was the story of the heritage of African Americans. Our anatomical and physiological roots are also a fascinating study. By examining these roots, we can better know ourselves for what we are, and we will discover a most wonderful story. The psalmist proclaimed in the Bible, "For thou didst form my inward parts, thou didst knit me together in my mother's womb . . . when I was being made in secret." This would suggest that there is a great deal to be learned about our roots and the way we are constructed. Truly we are made "in secret," for there is much we do not yet know about the processes of our development.

Many years of careful research have uncovered some of the body's secrets, but each discovery has begged for yet deeper investigation into the body's amazing structure and function. It is a biological axiom that structure is intimately related to function. Do you think it is important to have good bowel and digestive function? If so, you must pay attention to bowel structure, for, most assuredly, the first requirement of good function is good structure.

We have seen that digestive upsets and dysfunctions are among the most common health complaints. Is there a person who hasn't suffered from bad breath, upset stomach, cramps, headache, indigestion, or constipation at some time in his or her life? It is revealing that the over-the-counter medications used for these very complaints account for the largest sales volumes among nonprescription drugs. What is not so well known is what we are discussing here—namely, that problems in the digestive tract can cause symptoms to appear almost anywhere in the body, even in areas far removed from the bowel, such as the head and even the feet.

A NEW CONCEPTION

Our search for our physical roots begins with the moment of conception. On the physical plane, the new cell that is created by the union of sperm with egg begins immediately to divide to form two cells. Then, each newly formed cell repeats the division process until, after three or four days, a little ball of cells exists. Though microscopic, this ball of cells bears a striking resemblance to the common mulberry. At this stage, the tiny "mulberry" is composed of twelve to sixteen cells and is known as a morula, which, by the way, is Latin for "mulberry." By the end of the first week of its gestation, the embryo, now known as a zygote, is ready for implantation in the womb. There it will be nourished to term by the mother. A new person is on the way!

Near the end of the first month following conception, some fantastic events occur. The developing body assumes a cylindrical form. A groove soon appears and deepens, becoming the neural canal, which is the forerunner of the nervous system, including the brain and the spinal cord. The innermost layer of cells now rolls into a tube, called the primitive gut tube, which eventually becomes the digestive tract.

We can understand this early development more easily if we think of a tree. If your trees are like the ones in my back yard, they sometimes have an aesthetically displeasing but perfectly normal biological habit of sprouting little shoots almost anywhere along the trunk. Most people quickly trim off these little shoots, as they tend to mar the appearance of the tree. Left unattended, the shoots soon grow into branches. Before you trim the shoots off your tree the next time, notice that the bark of the tree trunk is contiguous with the bark covering the new shoots. The bark covering all of the limbs is literally an extension of the bark of the trunk. You see, the new limbs merely "bud out" from the trunk or from existing limbs.

If you would liken the primitive human intestinal tract to the trunk of a tree, you will find that many of our internal organs bud out from the gut tube in much the same way that young limbs bud out from the tree trunk. And, like the bark that covers the branches of the tree, none other than the intestinal wall itself surrounds and covers these organs. Figure 4.1 provides a clear-cut picture of this process. If you push your finger into the side of an inflated balloon, you will see immediately that your finger is surrounded or covered by the material of the balloon. In like manner, the liver is covered with intestinal wall as it buds out from the intestinal tube. The pancreas is also surrounded by intestinal wall. So are the gallbladder, the stomach, the lungs, and even the urinary bladder. How about the trachea, larynx, and pharynx? These, too! Each develops by budding out from the primitive gut tube, from the intestinal tract, assuming as its covering the intestinal wall complete with its supply of nerves.

The intestinal tract, along with its nerve supply, constitutes part of your roots, your early development, when you were being "made in secret." Now that you have been primed by this biology lesson, you are ready to see why we consider the bowel to be king and how the neural-arc reflex works.

A diverticulum acts as a trap, much like the curved pipes under a sink. It is prone to collecting debris that would be carried out with a normal bowel movement if the diverticulum were not there. I have

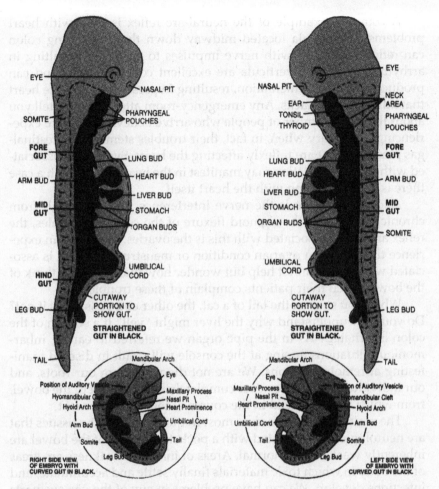

Figure 4.1. During the embryonic stage, the organs and limbs bud out from the bowel.

described this trapped material as being similar to the flotsam that collects at the bend of a stream, refuse that has been sidelined from the main current and is unable to move on. In like manner, colonic debris can collect in the bends and pockets of the bowel. In the moist, bacterially laden, warm body, this trapped material stagnates and ferments, becoming an irritant to the colon wall. The resultant nerve irritation sends messages via established nerve routes and reflexly affects distant locations. Thus it is that irritations in a particular segment of the bowel often are associated with symptoms in other areas of the body. Yet when people are treated for these symptoms, the bowel is almost never considered.

A common example of the neural-arc reflex is seen with heart problems. Diverticula located midway down the descending colon can reflexly interfere with nerve impulses to the heart, resulting in arrhythmias. Also, diverticula are excellent collection sites and can produce gas from fermentation, resulting in pressures upon the heart that mimic heart attacks. Any emergency-room attendant will tell you about the large number of people who arrive believing they are experiencing a coronary when, in fact, their troubles stem from intestinal-gas pressures that are reflexly affecting the heart. Symptoms associated with a bowel irritation may manifest in the heart, but in such a case there is nothing wrong with the heart itself.

Another example is the nerve interference that can result from chronic irritation at the sigmoid flexure of the colon. In females, the reflex area most associated with this is the ovaries. I know from experience that many an ovarian condition or menstrual problem is associated with this. I cannot help but wonder how many doctors think of the bowel when their patients complain of these troubles.

When you step on the tail of a cat, the other end yells, does it not? Do you now understand why the liver might "yell" if a section of the colon is irritated? As in the pipe organ we referred to earlier, inharmonious situations arising at the console will result in discord manifesting at remote locations. We are not divorced from our roots, and our individual organs are never completely independent of the bowel, from which they emerged in the course of their development.

The neural-arc reflex occurs most frequently when the tissues that are neurologically associated with a pocketed section of the bowel are inherently weaker than normal. Areas of inherent weakness are areas of the body in which toxic materials finally settle and accumulate, and infections develop. We can have problems in any of the various parts of the body, and invariably, these infections are induced by irritations or problems in the bowel due to the neural-arc reflex. In my studies over the last forty-five years, I have found a striking correlation between conditions in sections of the bowel and conditions in other specific parts of the body. For example, when a patient complains of a breast condition, there is a certain place in the bowel that I suspect harbors a low-grade infection that is affecting the breast area. The following cases further demonstrate the relationship.

WHAT THE DOCTOR SEES, BUT DOESN'T RECOGNIZE

Mrs. Jones is forty-seven. She is complaining of a stiff and painful left shoulder that she says has bothered her from time to time over the past several years. "It comes and goes," she states. "I have problems with it about twice a year. With treatment and pain medication, it relents and is good for six to eight months. Then it's back again." She asks why it recurs, stating that she is right-handed and can think of no abuse or trauma associated with her left shoulder. Continuing with the history-taking, we find that she has been to several doctors over the years and has received various types of treatment for the shoulder including injections of the steroid cortisone. All of the treatments reduced the acute symptoms, but none prevented the condition from returning.

Examination of this patient reveals tense and painful muscles associated with certain shoulder movements. There is a marked decrease in the range of normal movement of the arm and shoulder. She cannot raise her arm over her head on the affected side. Anything but minimal and cautious movements of her arm elicit immediate pain. Depending upon the particulars, a condition such as this would probably be diagnosed as bursitis or tendinitis. How about frozen shoulder or tenosynovitis? Perhaps just acute myositis. All of these are painful inflammations localized to the shoulder area. I am trying to show that the names given to a condition may reveal little or nothing about the condition's root cause or true location.

The preceding scenario occurs countless times in thousands of doctor's offices. The complaint usually takes the following form: There is a history of recurrence. The patient cannot think of any good reason why the problem should occur. He or she often cannot relate the condition to any injury, trauma, or strain. This type of situation is crying, "Look to the bowel!" The father of medicine, Hippocrates, knew about the neural-arc reflex. He reminded physicians that in every patient complaint, they should look not only to the spine, but also to the bowel.

Mrs. Jones was eventually treated through diet. She was also educated in the proper care of the bowel and embarked on a program of colon cleansing very similar to the one outlined in this book. It is particularly significant that no treatment was applied to the affected shoulder, the area of main complaint. The patient recovered completely and no longer suffers pain in her shoulder.

In another instance, a boy came to me with problems in his left leg. For three years, he had been receiving massage plus mechanical and chemical treatments. I refused to treat him until he had a barium X-ray series done. He had never had films of his lower GI tract taken. It was discovered that he had cancer of the sigmoid colon, and he died a few months later. It was my opinion at the time that his tumor had been causing a reflex condition in his leg, but he had been treated only for the leg problem. In thousands of cases of specific troubles in various organs of the body, I've been able to trace the cause to the bowel and verify the bowel troubles.

In Germany, for instance, I offered tissue cleansing at Dr. Martin's Sanitarium for Cellular Therapy. While at the sanitarium, I learned that Benjamin Gaylord Hauser, then one of the most popular lecturers in the United States, had just left. I was able to view the X-ray pictures of his bowel, which showed diverticula halfway down the descending colon. In my experience, I have found that diverticula in this location often indicate bronchial and lung trouble due to the neural-arc reflex. The doctors in Europe advised Mr. Hauser to seek my counsel concerning his bowel. Mr. Hauser did not see me, however, and shortly after returning to the United States to celebrate his ninetieth birthday, he came down with pneumonia and died. Had he known about the neural-arc reflex from his bowel to his bronchioles, he might have taken steps to improve his bowel condition, perhaps adding a few more years to his distinguished life.

I once examined a lady who suffered from an acute exacerbation of chronic torticollis (wry neck). In this condition, contracted neck muscles cause the head to be held in an unnatural position. When I examined her and told her that I would make a chiropractic adjustment to her neck, she refused. She related that she had received several neck adjustments, each of which seemed only to make the condition worse. She just couldn't stand to have anyone touch her neck again. Although as a chiropractor I'm "supposed" to make adjustments, and I was eager to practice my profession, I was also aware of the neural-arc reflex. When I asked if she ever had any bowel trouble, she indicated that she'd had problems for years. Lately, about the time the neck problem became acute, her bowel had become worse. Instead of performing an adjustment, I advised the lady to immediately take an enema. She had three enemas within one hour, and while I was still there, she obtained complete relief from her stiff and painful neck. This was quite an eye-opening experience, one that I have not forgotten in all these years.

Another situation that dramatically illustrates the neural-arc reflex was related to me by Dr. Bodeen. He and his wife, Joyce, who oversees the tissue-cleansing program for his patients, brought to my attention a woman who had lost her voice. Able to speak only in a whisper, the woman stated that this condition occurred periodically for no apparent reason and would last from days to weeks. In this case again, she could not relate it to any sickness, event, or trauma. The situation was further complicated by the fact that she was employed in Canada as a telephone operator!

This patient revealed that she had spent much time and money seeking the best doctors in an effort to determine the reasons for these mysterious episodes. When a number of doctors could give no satisfactory physical reason for her periodic loss of voice, it was suggested that she see a psychiatrist. Her doctor thought it could be an emotional problem. Nobody likes to hear this from a doctor. I have personally seen many people in my office who, with great emotion, tearfully begged me not to tell them their problems were merely the result of some psychological disturbance, as their doctors had condescendingly suggested. This is not to say that some persons do not have genuine psychological problems or that physical disease is not without its psychological and emotional aspects and vice versa. But surely, it is not good practice to write off what is essentially a physical condition as an emotional problem merely because it eludes the doctor's diagnostic acumen. This practice causes untold mental suffering in misdiagnosed patients, of which this woman was one.

I am pleased to tell you that on the third day of the tissue-cleansing program, the woman regained her voice. In fact, her voice was once again strong and clear. Regaining her voice brought happiness enough, but it was most satisfying to her to learn that she had experienced the symptom due to a direct relationship with a colon problem. It was a classic manifestation of the neural-arc reflex. Her doctors had been quite correct in declaring they could find no problem with her vocal apparatus. A problem in the bowel was causing the symptoms in a distant but neurologically related area. To date, this patient has not had a return of her symptoms. Neither her throat nor vocal cords were treated. No medications of any kind were administered. Colon cleansing was the only treatment.

This case and all the others described here should impress upon you the importance of the neural-arc reflex and the variety of conditions in which it may be involved. This is why we say that the bowel is king, out of respect for the myriad problems that can be related to dysfunctions of the digestive tract.

Do you think the bowel can affect your liver? Your kidneys? How about your feet? The bowel can affect anything. And I mean anything. Anywhere. Anytime. People are suffering from conditions they would never in their wildest dreams think could have anything to do with the bowel. These people are usually treated for the symptoms of their condition rather than for the cause of their distress. Now I want to tell you why.

NO PAIN NERVES, NO PAIN

Pain is the one thing that brings most people to the doctor. It takes a certain type of nerve to transmit what is interpreted by the brain as pain. Although there are millions of nerves in the body, only some transmit pain information. In fact, the brain itself has no pain sensors. It seems odd that the organ which interprets certain nerve impulses as pain has no capacity to receive pain sensations from its own structure. It's like the proverbial shoemaker who has no shoes to wear on his own feet! In fact, surgeons find there is no pain or other feeling elicited when the brain is touched or even cut! Did you know that the same is true of the bowel? Bowel surgery requires anesthetic so that the surgeon can cut through the muscular abdominal wall, which is pain-sensitive. Once inside the abdominal cavity, the surgeon may handle the bowel, both large and small, without causing pain.

Now you should begin to see why people can have problems in the bowel, even of long standing, and frequently experience no pain there. It is not uncommon for people to have severe problems, even bleeding, in the bowel and experience no pain or discomfort at the site. Yet, as we are now aware, there may be, and usually are, problems manifesting at a secondary and distant site that is reflexly stimulated by a primary bowel condition. And there may be intense pain at the secondary site with no discomfort whatsoever at the primary site, the bowel. This is why we say that by the time a person experiences localized bowel pain, the condition is often very serious and in need of immediate attention.

Even though the bowel is greatly lacking in pain-receptor nerves when compared to other parts of the body, people can and do experience symptoms in the bowel. The problem is that the early symptoms are so ordinary, they usually do not receive serious attention. They are let go. It is not unusual for people to neglect tell-tale digestive symptoms for months or even years. This provides time for intestinal problems to become quite deep-seated and chronic. During this time, remote sites are likely to become disturbed via the neural-arc reflex. Something as simple as recurring bouts of indigestion, chronic constipation, gastritis (stomach inflammation), or ulcers can be the alarm signal that all is not well in the digestive area. Although these conditions may be early warning signals, most people will, unfortunately, just medicate their symptoms, choosing from a vast array of over-the-counter nostrums available at the local pharmacy. Is it any wonder that laxatives and pain relievers are the largest selling over-the-counter medications?

Often when there are symptoms that require treatment, a particular organ of the body is treated even though the bowel is the source of the problem. Consider the string of events leading to the death of John Wayne. Oftentimes, busy people such as celebrities, who must eat out a good deal and be on the move almost constantly, have difficulty finding the time to eat properly. They do not eat the right foods in a calm, pleasant, unrushed manner in an attractive environment. We might think of eating habits when we consider all of Wayne's operations together. His first operation was for cancer of the lungs. His second operation was for cancer of the stomach. But his third and last operation was for cancer of the bowel. Is it possible that he should have been treated for a bowel condition long before any problems arose in the stomach and lungs? I wonder how his bowel health was before any cancer was detected.

Another famous entertainer, comedian Jack Benny, had a "perfect" examination just two months before he died of cancer. I don't know whether or not he had a barium study or other examination of the digestive tract, especially the colon. I do know that the most common places for cancer of the bowel are the sigmoid colon and the lower portion of the ascending colon. It would have been good to check these places. As you become more "bowel-minded," these thoughts will come to your mind. And as you become bowel-minded, you can learn to break the patterns that might otherwise prove fatal.

BREAKING THE NEURAL-ARC REFLEX

Neural-arc-reflex activity is not only genetic in origin, but is the cumulative result of years of bad habits. Everyone knows that a bad habit is difficult to break. The only way to break a bad habit is to replace it with a good habit. Physiologically speaking, replacement therapy involves the body's replacing old tissue with new. This happens when, through nutrition, we replace the chemical elements that we have been lacking in the body. Replacement therapy also applies to the mental side of life when we practice a better way of living. Working to cultivate a good habit to overcome a destructive one is a type of replacement therapy.

The nervous system sees no difference between a good habit and a bad one. Physiologically, they are both established in the same way. Because good habits, thankfully, are as tenacious as bad ones, good habits serve us well our entire lives. I've never heard anybody complain about a good habit! Even though all habits take time to become established, there is no time like the present to begin practicing good ones. Procrastination serves only to foster undesirable habits by providing additional time for them to become entrenched.

Everyone knows that if you learn a piece of music with the wrong timing or a few wrong notes, you have an extremely difficult time unlearning it. We may spend hours learning to correct our mistakes, but if we become fatigued or do not pay close attention to the task, we habitually slide back into those old mistakes. So it is with the neural-arc reflex.

The best way to break the path of the neural-arc reflex is with the program outlined in this book. The Ultimate Tissue Cleansing Program presented here is a powerful adjunct in establishing good habits to replace old destructive ones. This program, combined with the essentials of proper diet and a healthy lifestyle, will help prevent the habitual symptoms associated with a destructive neural-arc reflex. Used regularly as directed, the program will break the cycle of referred symptoms by taking care of the problem at its source—the bowel. To take care of the kingdom, we must first take care of the king! Let us now learn about the program that puts us on the path to a cleaner and healthier bowel and normalizes the aberrant neural-arc reflex.

EMOTIONS AND THE BOWEL

We have seen how the neural-arc reflex operates and how nerve pathways can be established and facilitated from the bowel to other areas of the body. Now we must consider the neural-arc reflex in reverse. Our emotions—that is, our feelings and mental state—have a great effect on the bowel, so much so that the bowel in ancient times was called "the seat of the emotions." Everyone knows that, although the emotions may have an effect upon the heart, it is much more common to need toilet facilities than a cardiologist when the emotions are accentuated.

The colon is extremely sensitive and is influenced greatly by every emotion, both positive and negative. It has been proven that unpleasant emotions can interfere with the peristalsis of the colon, regardless of how slight the excitement, anxiety, or apprehension is. This is because the brain sends as well as receives nerve impulses. Until now, we have merely considered how nerve impulses coming *from* the bowel can affect other parts of the body, but there are also nerves going *to* the bowel.

Anatomically, the nerves tend to follow the paths of the blood vessels. They innervate the blood vessels, constricting or dilating them, as the case may be, as well as having a contracting or relaxing effect, or an irritating or soothing effect, upon the tissues in which they terminate. Thus, every emotion mediated via the nervous system has an effect upon the blood supply and the muscles of the colon. Our state of mind—that is, our thoughts—can facilitate the neural-arc reflex, especially at the points in the bowel where there are inherent tissue weaknesses. This is the neural-arc reflex in reverse.

Fear and anxiety can have profound effects, for the tensed colon may respond with diarrhea or constipation as the nerve impulses carry the message of fright to the bowel. The bowel remains affected until the apprehension or fear subsides. One study that included X-rays of dogs and cats clearly showed the effects and associations of certain emotions on the nervous system and the colon. The dogs, placed in unfamiliar surroundings, ceased to have peristalsis in the colon for several hours. When the cats' tails were pinched, peristalsis ceased until the cats were once again contented. On the other hand, battlefront surgeons are familiar with the loss of bladder and bowel control experienced by soldiers exposed to the stress and terror of battle conditions. Peristalsis can be triggered as well as halted by emotionally impacting events.

Anger and grief may cause the bowel to stop secreting and contracting, both of which are necessary for good digestion and for the evacuation of wastes from the body. I, therefore, recommend that my patients not eat when they are upset or excited. In the same vein, I also advise them to be careful never to let their table conversations be such that they become emotional or upset while consuming their meals. Stress has no place at the dinner table.

Certain common bowel disorders are known to be linked to the mental side of being. It is known that colitis, for example, has to do as much with the thoughts and emotions as with the bowel. In fact, it has been clinically affirmed that nearly all functional bowel disorders have a definite mental counterpart. Inflammation of the bowel can be exacerbated and even brought on by nervous tension and stress.

People have much better bowel movements when they are free of emotional pain and financial worry. Good companionship, relaxation, and music can be stress-reducing and relaxing, and thus conducive to good bowel movements. The bowel has to be taken care of through the holistic healing arts, rather than by some medication, adjustment, reflex-therapy treatment, or even diet. Each of these will bring some improvement, but the bowel will not function correctly until we learn how to live properly. There is a right way of living, and it isn't just food and diet. It is important to approve of yourself and to get along with other people, because when it comes to the bowel, it isn't always *what* is wrong with you. It may be *who* is wrong with you!

Chapter 5

The Seven-Day Cleansing Program

I n previous chapters I pointed out that an underactive toxic bowel invites disease in three ways. First, it creates in itself a highly reactive, disease-friendly environment. Second, its slower transit time allows more toxic substances to penetrate the bowel wall and pass into the blood and lymph. From here, they spread throughout the body, creating a greater vulnerability to disease in tissues already weakened by other means. Third, any inflammations that develop activate the neural-arc reflex, causing symptoms in remote parts of the body.

There is also a fourth way an underactive toxic bowel opens the door to disease. When the amount of toxic material increases in the body, as its does when bowel transit time is slowed, the immune system soon becomes depressed. It takes a lot of white blood cells to get rid of the toxic debris in the system, leaving few to defend the body against the various types of microorganisms that cause disease. Cancer and many other degenerative diseases develop more readily when the body's immune system is depressed.

The most effective response to all the disease-inviting consequences of an underactive toxic bowel is to cleanse the bowel as thoroughly as possible. The immune system can be built up only in a clean body, a body with a minimal amount of accumulated toxic material. The presence of significant quantities of toxic material in the tissues means that the body's natural defenses have been compromised or even overcome. Health is restored by cleansing the tissues through improved management and care of all the elimination systems, especially the bowel. This must be followed by a healthier lifestyle that

101

includes an improved diet, exercise, fresh air, sunshine, and a positive outlook on life. In my complete bowel-cleansing program, as set forth in this book, exceptional improvements have been observed and recorded.

As the methods presented in the following pages are further understood and tested, I hope to find them used in hospitals and sanitariums in the treatment of various disease conditions. Please remember that the Ultimate Tissue Cleansing Program is designed to be part of a preventive-healthcare system in which the results of bad habits may begin to be reversed. Good results with lasting quality will not be evident as long as destructive habits are continued.

This program is for the person who wants to work and is willing to start anew. Going into the Ultimate Tissue Cleansing Program, you must have a new mindset. Sowing and cultivating life-generating practices and forsaking destructive, health-destroying ones mark a new beginning that will ultimately enable you to reap the harvest of renewed health and vitality.

The Ultimate Tissue Cleansing Program uses mechanical, dietary, and lifestyle techniques to rid the body of accumulated toxic materials. The program lasts six to eight months and includes the following six steps:

1. Follow the Seven-Day Cleansing Program.

2. Follow the Seven-Week Building and Replacement Program.

3. Repeat the Seven-Day Cleansing Program.

4. Repeat the Seven-Week Building and Replacement Program.

5. Continue cycling through the cleansing program and the building program for a period of six to eight months.

6. Return to a regular, wholesome diet.

The Ultimate Tissue Cleansing Program may be repeated as needed. Before beginning the program, you may wish to consult with your healthcare provider.

Although there are many therapeutic approaches to restoring and maintaining health today, the presence of toxic settlements in the body prevents most of these methods from being completely successful. If a treatment does not work toward complete detoxification, the replacement of tissues will not take place as it should. The complete rebuilding process involves the replacement of old, underactive tissue with new, clean, efficiently working tissue. Many kinds of processes can be used to alleviate a chronic or degenerative condition, but natural therapeutics and right living are the best. The wise doctor will, when possible, choose a natural and drug-free method that steers clear of the harmful suppression of symptoms as well as damaging side effects.

The finest and quickest way that I know to detoxify the body begins with the bowel. Because the bowel is the king of all the elimination systems, it is wise to start any detoxification program by cleansing the bowel and returning it to proper function. Furthermore, many people do not take care of their bowel as they should. An improper diet, pressured lifestyle, and failure to heed nature's call all contribute to common bowel dysfunction. The Ultimate Tissue Cleansing Program is a special method of cleansing the bowel, utilizing water and natural supplements and additives, so that normal bowel function can be resumed. Of course, this program is no substitute for proper diet and certain lifestyle changes that may be necessary in order to maintain a healthy bowel and enjoy the optimum function that nature intended.

THE MINDSET FOR TISSUE CLEANSING

Before making any physical preparations for the Ultimate Tissue Cleansing Program, it is essential to consider mental readiness. Not every person has the mindset necessary for accepting all the potential benefits. It is now time to resolve to change some key things rooted in your past such as negative attitudes, improper dietary habits, and wrongful living in general. Over the years, your bowel has probably not been fed properly and has been underactive. It is now time to get rid of all the unnecessary accumulations it is housing.

When you go through the Ultimate Tissue Cleansing Program, you will see things you'll find hard to accept. You don't yet realize what can come out of the bowel. After just one cleansing session, I've seen as much as three gallons of hard, toxic material come from one person. It's almost unbelievable. I've seen grape seeds expelled from the bowel of a person who declared that he had not eaten any grapes for nine months. Where had these grape seeds been? I've seen popcorn come out of a person who hadn't eaten popcorn for three years. Where had it been? We accumulate these things in the mucous membrane that lines the bowel. This mucous membrane can hold toxic material nestled in its folds for a very long time. I never believed the intestinal tract could be so loaded with mucus, so black and so toxic, but I had the chance to see this while on the cleansing program myself.

We will soon look at the means of breaking down the heavy mucous membrane lining the colon, but first we must consider how the colon accumulates this much of a buildup. The intestinal tract secretes mucus as a protection against irritation. When ingested material (food) irritates the bowel or is not digested properly and leaves irritating residues, the bowel's natural response is to secrete mucus in order to protect its delicate tissues. The colon builds up this mucus in much the same way an oyster creates a pearl to protect its delicate tissues from a sharp grain of sand. When the bowel contents are sluggish and slow-moving, the irritation is compounded.

Donald J. Mantell, M.D., said, "I believe that the colon is one of the areas most neglected by the medical establishment." He went on to comment, "It is quite interesting to see what is expelled during a normal colonic treatment. One may see mucus, parasites, and very old feculent material that may have been living in the patient's colon for years. It looks like vulcanized rubber, and has that kind of consistency." This feculent material and other results of the Ultimate Tissue Cleansing Program are shown on pages 213 through 222. *Warning: This material is rather graphic in nature and you may not wish to view it.*

A number of people have passed parasites during the seven-day cleanse. One woman passed "a bucket of worms." Another found her breast problems relieved by the elimation of parasites, reminding us again of the reflex relationship of the bowel to all the parts of the body.

More and more authorities today are recognizing that a clean colon is necessary for good health. As we have seen, disorders such as appendicitis; an infected liver, gallbladder, and tonsils; dysfunction of the heart and blood vessels; sinusitis; arthritis; and rheumatism no doubt have their origins in a sluggish colon. An increasing number of morbid conditions in the flexures of the colon, the rectum, and the anus are being realized. Consider the amount of surgery and the various therapies performed today for hemorrhoids, fistulas (abnormal ducts), prostate disturbances, and malignancies. If you have read this far, you should no longer have any doubt in your mind about the relation between the condition of the intestinal tract and the health of the rest of the body. Intestinal management is probably the most important thing a person can learn as part of a total health-building routine. Let us, therefore, begin our preparations for the Ultimate Tissue Cleansing Program.

Many supplies—both consumable and permanent—are needed for the first phase of the cleansing program. A complete "Checklist of Tools and Supplies for the Seven-Day Cleansing Program" can be found on page 105. Descriptions of the supplies along with explanations of their

Checklist of Tools and Supplies for the Seven-Day Cleansing Program

A number of tools, supplies, food items, and supplements are needed for the Seven-Day Cleansing Program. In the list of foods and supplements, the total amount of each item that may be utilized during the cleansing program is listed. Not everyone uses the same amount of each item, and many of the items are packaged in different amounts by the different manufacturers. When shopping for these items, read the labels to determine which size packages are the best for you. Additional items will be needed for the Seven-Week Building and Replacement Program.

The basic list of items needed for the Seven-Day Cleansing Program is as follows:

❏ Tools

- Colema board with attachments
- Plastic rectal tip
- Sturdy chair or stool for supporting the head of the colema board (optional)
- 4- to 5-gallon plastic bucket
- Spigot for the bucket (optional)
- Towel for cushioning your back on the colema board (optional)
- Pillow for cushioning your head on the colema board (optional)
- Infant rectal syringe
- Long-handled natural-bristle brush for skin brushing
- Empty 1-pint jar with a tight lid for the Cleansing Drink
- Tennis ball for massaging your abdomen during the colema (optional)

❑ Supplies
- 1 quart of Neolife Rugged Red germicidal solution
- One 3.75-ounce tube of K-Y lubricating jelly

❑ Foods and Supplements
- 35 tablespoons of apple cider vinegar for the Cleansing Drink
- 70 ounces of apple juice for the Cleansing Drink
- 28 tablespoons of liquid calcium-magnesium, 320 milligrams of calcium and 40 milligrams of magnesium per ounce
- 480 tablets of chlorella, 200 milligrams per tablet, or 224 tablets of alfalfa, 550 milligrams per tablet
- 24 teaspoons of liquid chlorophyll, 140 milligrams per ounce
- Additional liquid chlorophyll for the colemas (optional)
- 35 tablespoons of clay water for the Cleansing Drink
- Additional clay water for the colemas (optional)
- 14 gelatin capsules of cod liver oil, 2,500 IU (international units) of vitamin A and 270 IU of vitamin D per capsule
- 152 tablets of digestive-enzyme supplement
- 28 tablets of dulse, 550 milligrams per tablet
- 14 tablespoons of flaxseed
- Additional flaxseed for flaxseed tea and the colemas (optional)
- Garlic cloves for the colemas (optional)
- 2 tablets of herbal laxative
- Herbal tea
- 35 teaspoons of raw honey for the Cleansing Drink
- 35 rounded teaspoons of intestinal cleanser for the Cleansing Drink
- Fruit and/or vegetable juice
- 92 tablets of niacin, 50 milligrams per tablet
- 1 cup of olive oil
- 176 tablets of vitamin C, 100 milligrams per tablet

- Water for the colemas, drinks, and broths, and to dilute the liquid chlorophyll
- 28 gelatin capsules of wheat germ oil, approximately 500 milligrams per capsule
- 56 tablets of whole beet juice concentrate, approximately 300 milligrams per capsule

For descriptions of these items and their uses, read this entire chapter.

---

uses are provided in the following pages. Mail-order sources are provided in Appendix B. For the supplies needed for the Seven-Week Building and Replacement Program, see Chapter 6.

SUPPLEMENTS

The following supplements are used in the Seven-Day Cleansing Program for specific reasons. So that you may more fully appreciate the usefulness of these items, I present here brief explanations of their properties. Information about selected suppliers appears in Appendix B.

Alfalfa

Alfalfa tablets contain all the fiber material from the stems and leaves of the alfalfa plant. This fiber acts as a bulk and a material that a ballooned or weakened bowel can work against to develop improved tone. This encourages a faster transit time. I use this supplement for practically every patient who needs to build bowel tone. Although alfalfa offers the proper bulk, it sometimes produces more gas when a lazy bowel is stirred. For this reason, I sometimes use a couple of digestive-enzyme tablets along with the alfalfa to help get rid of the gas. Alfalfa is also a natural source of silicon and chlorophyll.

Apple Cider Vinegar

High in potassium, apple cider vinegar is good for relieving any mucous or catarrhal conditions. It helps alkalinize the system, provides needed nutrients for muscle tissue, and helps prevent elec-

trolyte depletion. I do not recommend distilled white vinegar, which
is not a natural product.

Apple Juice

Apple juice is very good for the bowel because it is high in pectin,
which is a moisture-holding substance. It is also a good source of
potassium and other electrolytes. Apple juice may have a slight laxative effect in some people. Unfiltered, unprocessed apple juice is best,
if you can obtain it.

Calcium-Magnesium

Combination calcium-magnesium supplements come in various
forms, but I prefer the liquid. Look for a colloidal suspension of calcium, magnesium, phosphorus, and manganese in pure demineralized
water. Calcium and magnesium are vital for muscle contraction and
relaxation, so important in good bowel action and tone.

Chlorella

Chlorella is a highly nutritious, single-celled algae that contains a
greater percentage of chlorophyll than any other product. Because of
this, I believe it is the best detoxifier known. Several brands of chlorella are currently on the market. One is manufactured by a Japanese
company that developed a patented process in which the cell wall of
the chlorella is fractionated, making it easier for the product to be
assimilated by the body. I toured a Japanese chlorella facility several
years ago and authored the book *Chlorella: Gem of the Orient*.

Clay Water

Clay water is a colloidal suspension of clay in water, with the clay particles so fine that they cannot be separated out. Clay water is not an
absorbent, but rather a magnet, attracting to itself many undesirable
chemicals. Some kinds of clay particles can adsorb (incorporate into
their surface) forty times their own weight in toxic substances. One
brand of clay water that I have found to work well is Bentonite Clay
Water (Vit-Ra-Tox Number 16) by V.E. Irons, Inc. Bentonite, also
known as montmorillnite, is a specific type of clay first discovered
near Fort Benton, Wyoming.

Cod Liver Oil

Cod liver oil provides lubrication for the bowel and stimulates the gallbladder to contract and release bile. It is an excellent source of vitamins A and D, which are needed for good elimination. Norwegian cod liver oil is best.

Digestive-Enzyme Supplement

Digestive-enzyme supplement is a mixture of digestive enzymes that help bring down the mucous lining of the digestive tract. The digestive-enzyme supplement used on the Seven-Day Cleansing Program should contain pancreatin concentrate from animal sources. Digestive-enzyme supplement is very powerful, loosening the mucous lining in preparation for its removal during the seven-day cleanse. A good product is Enzymatic Supplement, also known as Vit-Ra-Tox Number 54, manufactured by V.E. Irons, Inc.

Dulse

Also known as kelp, dulse quickens the action of the thyroid gland and speeds up the metabolism, causing the blood to circulate better. Dulse is seaweed, which contains natural, organic iodine, never to be confused with chemical, inorganic iodine, which is poisonous. *Never use medicinal iodine as a substitute for dulse.* Dulse comes in tablet form. Nova Scotia dulse from cold northern waters is deemed best.

Flaxseed

Flaxseed is an excellent bulk-maker. In extreme cases of ulcerated colitis or other bowel irritations or inflammations, it is a soothing and healing emollient when put into the colema water in the form of a decoction or tea. It is also a good bowel lubricant. You can add a teaspoon or more of liquid chlorophyll to the flaxseed tea to be used in the colema water.

Flaxseed tea can be taken orally as well. (For a recipe, see page 120.) If you take it orally, drink one cup of the tea with one teaspoon of liquid chlorophyll three times a day. Flaxseed tea taken orally can be used in cases of extreme gas, spastic conditions, colitis, and the like. I have never found anyone who could not take flaxseed tea, either as a health drink or an enema.

Garlic

Nothing can live in garlic! Because intestinal parasites find garlic most disagreeable, it is used to help rid the intestine of established parasites. I recommend its use in the Ultimate Tissue Cleansing Program just in case there is some parasitic infection.

Herbal Laxative Tablets

While no laxative should be taken on a regular basis, an herbal laxative taken as recommended on this tissue-cleansing program is not only safe, but beneficial. Make sure the product you buy contains an extract of cascara sagrada and aloe curacao herbs. All stimulative laxatives are habit-forming and are not for long-term use. Never get into a laxative habit.

Honey

Honey is used in the Cleansing Drink (see page 118) that is ingested daily during the Seven-Day Cleansing Program. There are lots of brands on the market, but be sure to obtain a honey that is raw and unheated—that is, that has not been heated to high temperatures or processed in any way that would alter it. Honey that is unheated and raw will proudly display this information on the label.

Intestinal Cleanser

The best intestinal cleansers are vegetable psyllium-seed products that come from the Near East. When mixed with water or another liquid, they form a mucilaginous bulk that holds moisture very well. The product attaches itself to the mucous lining of the colon, making it soft and loose so that it will move away from the bowel wall. Being a moisture-laden bulk, it helps the bowel achieve better peristaltic action.

A good intestinal cleanser is very important to the success of the tissue-cleansing program. Many psyllium products, especially those produced by pharmaceutical companies, do not include the husks and may also contain a significant amount of sugar. Be sure to read the label of any product you consider buying.

Liquid Chlorophyll

Before antibiotics came into common use, medical doctors sometimes used liquid chlorophyll diluted with sterile water to clean out deep surgical wounds, even severely infected ones. Chlorophyll used on infected wounds eliminates the foul odor associated with infection. Unlike antibiotics, chlorophyll is a probiotic, a friendly bacteria that makes conditions in the bowel inhospitable for undesirable bacteria. (For a discussion of probiotics, see page 137.) Liquid chlorophyll is available with or without added mint flavor. For colon cleansing, I suggest the unflavored type.

Niacin

A component of the vitamin-B complex, niacin produces a warm red flush and is used to push blood deep into underactive tissues so that they can be strengthened with vital nutrients. The symptoms of heat and flush are usually more or less confined to the head and upper extremities, and last from ten to twenty minutes. Adjust your niacin dose to the point where this flush is noticeable, but not severe. Some people react to niacin more strongly than others. Those who haven't taken niacin before should be careful with the first dose. Start with a small amount, say 25 milligrams, and work up to the point of a mild flush. When you're fasting or take niacin without food, it usually produces a stronger reaction. Always use niacin, not niacinamide, as the latter will not produce the same results.

Vitamin C

While the body is being purged of toxins and putrefactive material during the Seven-Day Cleansing Program, vitamin C helps protect it from new pollutants. Although any quality vitamin C can be used, be sure to obtain one that contains bioflavonoids and/or rutin to enhance the absorption of the vitamin. You see, vitamin C has been chemically determined to be ascorbic acid. As such, it can be easily and cheaply made in a laboratory. But without bioflavonoids or rutin, it is not a whole product and will not perform as well.

Wheat Germ Oil

Wheat germ oil is a cold-pressed oil containing no artificial colorings, preservatives, or flavorings. It is an excellent source of the essential fatty acids and vitamin E. Most of the time, the germ, the innermost portion of the wheat kernel, is removed from food during processing.

Because the germ is so often excluded from flour and other common products, we must get it from supplements.

Whole Beet Juice Concentrate

Whole beet juice concentrate contains concentrated dried beet juice from the whole plant. It is slightly laxative and has a cleansing effect on the liver. Raw shredded beet should be used for these reasons when off the Ultimate Tissue Cleansing Program.

FOR VEGETARIANS

Strict vegetarians often inquire about the need to use the few animal products employed on this regimen. Personally, I feel that the benefits of the regimen outweigh the negatives of using the animal products, especially since such a small amount of animal products is used and for such a brief period of time. Once the bowel is healthy again, the use of these substances can often be discontinued.

FOR ALLERGIC INDIVIDUALS

If you suffer an allergic reaction to any product recommended for use on the Seven-Day Cleansing Program, omit it from the regimen and seek counsel regarding an appropriate substitution. Sometimes an allergic reaction to a particular item will not become manifest until a later time, after some cleansing has been accomplished.

THE COLEMA APPARATUS

A colema is a special kind of enema that is more thorough in its internal cleansing of the bowel. It takes slightly longer, uses more water, and involves special dietary procedures that make the cleansing deep and powerful, yet very safe. A colema requires special equipment and is generally more comfortable than an enema.

A colema board, shown in Figure 5.1, is an essential component of the Ultimate Tissue Cleansing Program. The board is designed to allow the user to comfortably recline during the cleanse. The board consists of a piece of fiberglass or plastic-covered wood about fifteen inches wide and four feet long. Note that the board is supported on each end to make it capable of holding the weight of a person. It has a hole in one end that is placed over the toilet. The other end is supported by a chair that is just an inch or two higher than the toilet,

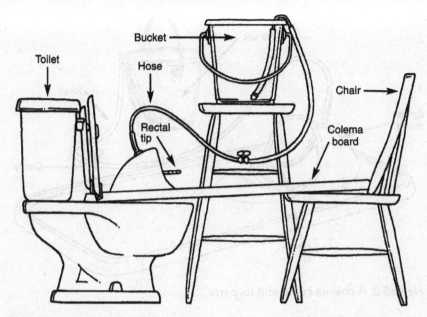

Figure 5.1. A colema board.

causing the board to incline slightly. This helps direct the flow of the bowel waste into the toilet.

A four- to five-gallon plastic bucket is hung above the board. A hose uses gravity to transport water from the bucket to a small-diameter plastic tip that is partially inserted into the rectum. The pencil-sized plastic tip remains in the rectum as the colema solution and the toxic waste material pass around it, allowing elimination to take place without the necessity of getting up to sit on the toilet. During the entire colema, the water need not be shut off (although it may be, at the user's convenience), nor the tip removed. Not having to remove the tip is one of the main differences between the colema and the enema. The water flows in and the toxic waste matter comes out and is directed immediately into the toilet. When the colema solution in the five-gallon bucket is gone, usually in about one-half hour, the procedure, explained and illustrated on page 117, is complete. During the Seven-Day Cleansing Program, colemas are taken once in the morning and once at night.

The colema board and its associated parts, illustrated in Figure 5.2, are a major advance for those interested in becoming involved in their own healing process. The equipment is lightweight, relatively inexpensive, easily stored, portable, and very effective. Not only does

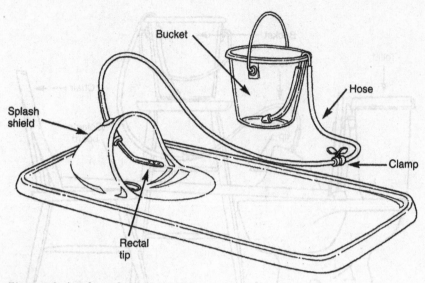

Figure 5.2. A colema board and its parts.

it make a colon treatment possible at home, but it also makes it easier to plan your own routine, saving both time and money. Perhaps best of all, the process leaves you in complete control. You are the sole operator of the colema, requiring no attendant. You have the advantage of convenience, simplicity, and complete privacy.

There are now several manufacturers of boards for tissue cleansing. I have tried a number of boards, but tend to prefer those from Colema Boards of California, Inc., which are available in one-piece or folding models. Although more expensive, the folding model has the advantage of greater portability and will fit in a suitcase for traveling. Other brands of boards have a slightly different design, are constructed of various materials, and have different advantages and disadvantages. Some people make their own boards, preferring to save on the expense or to customize the board to better fit their particular needs.

Cautions and Considerations

Although I feel the colema is one of the most natural ways of putting water into the bowel and eliminating it without any extreme distention or problems, you need to make sure that you have no conditions that may present risks, mentally or physically. These include an obstruction in the bowel, a severe inflammatory condition, ulceration, and diverticulitis. If you have pressure or bleeding in the bowel, you should not take a colema. In addition, if you have trouble releasing the water once it has been inserted, you should skip the treatment. I do not recommend the program for persons with serious heart conditions unless they are supervised by a professional qualified to handle cardiac emergencies. People who have diabetes, tuberculosis, cancer, asthma, and other extreme degenerative diseases must also have guidance, sanction, and assistance from a capable health professional. Insulin-dependent diabetics need particular care, as their insulin needs may change dramatically during a fast and cleanse such as this.

Before beginning the cleansing program, you would be prudent to have a complete physical examination including blood and urine tests. Your examination should include a complete blood count (CBC), a protein-bound iodine (PBI) test, a serum multiple analysis consisting of twenty-four tests (SMA-24), an acid-alkaline fecal test, a test for fecal acidophilus bacteria, X-rays (if needed), and any other test that can be used to show the chemical, tissue, and functional changes brought about by the program. If you have any organ or system with a weakness or dysfunction, you should have it checked often. You may also find it advisable to have a barium X-ray study (upper and lower GI) to check for any conditions that might make the cleanse inappropriate. A barium study requires a doctor's prescription. If necessary, delay the cleanse until you can undertake it safely.

If you suffer from any serious bowel condition or wonder whether your health is good enough to take a colema, consult a physician. Obtain reasonable assurance from your physician that a bowel cleansing of this type will not produce negative effects in your particular case.

Many physicians do not understand the bowel-cleansing process nor its significance. They may respond to your intention to take a colema with anything from apathy to utter disdain. If possible, find a physician who approves of your taking an active role in your own health care. If you have severe toxic bowel, having the cooperation of your physician would be invaluable.

During the tissue cleanse, you should *not* discontinue taking any medications prescribed for certain symptoms or conditions. Be aware, however, that fasting and cleansing often cause medications to act more powerfully. Also, following the cleanse, your dosage may need to be adjusted (usually lowered). Occasionally, a medication may be entirely eliminated. If you take a medication, ask your prescribing physician for any special instructions.

If you have arthritis, you may have problems getting on and off the colema board. Also, the rheumatic acids in your body may be stirred up before being eliminated and before your body can be supplied with supplemental organic minerals. If your arthritis pain is acute, start off the first day of the program with a colema to help relieve the symptoms, then take the recommended supplements.

Should you experience any nausea during the colema, stop the water flow by closing the clamp on the hose. It often helps to use some pillows to prop yourself up a bit until the nausea fades. As you pass some of the water and waste material out of your colon, you should feel the nausea lessen. Then you can continue with your colema.

Frequent colonic irrigation, such as this program entails, may adversely affect the electrolyte balance of the colon. Electrolyte leaching is not desirable. The best way to avoid such leaching is to replenish the electrolyte minerals and lactobacillus organisms. The Ultimate Tissue Cleansing Program assures this replacement. Therefore, do not deviate from the directions given unless advised to do so by your doctor. I have never heard complaints from anyone who followed the precautions and directions in this book. Do not deviate from the regimen described in this book unless instructed to do so by your physician.

Ensure Sanitary Conditions

Throughout this book I stress the importance of internal cleanliness as the vehicle by which health is regained and maintained. The degree to which the colon is inhabited by harmful bacteria, parasites, and other organisms and substances varies greatly among individuals. What one person is able to hold in the bowel without obvious negative effects may be hazardous to another. Therefore, when engaging in the tissue-cleansing effort, you must exercise certain precautions to prevent the transference of any harmful bacteria or parasites. Contamination of one individual by another must be carefully avoided. This can best be accomplished by ensuring that each person has his or her own colema board and rectal tip.

Never allow another person to use your colema board unless the equipment has been completely sterilized. Microscopic organisms are very easily transferred to the colon by the use of an unclean rectal tip. After each colema, wash the plastic tip in warm soapy water, rinse it well under running water, and then immerse it in a germicidal solution such as Rugged Red by Neolife. Do not boil the plastic tip or place it in an alcohol solution. When not in use, the tip should be stored right in a bottle of germicidal solution.

To help prevent infection, sterilize the connector tube, the small section of tube that holds the rectal tip, before each use. The manufacturers of this apparatus have endeavored to make this system as easy as possible to keep clean by keeping it uncomplicated. The board must be thoroughly washed after each use to prevent contamination. It is very important that you adhere to this instruction for your health and well-being. Never be lax in this regard. Here, the old axiom, "Cleanliness is next to godliness," certainly applies.

One of the many advantages of the colema-board design is that there is no reverse flow of colonic debris through the colema tubing. This is one of the features that sets the colema apparatus apart from nearly all the other commercially available colonic-irrigation equipment. Because of this, the likelihood of contamination is greatly reduced. Even so, it is a good idea to occasionally cleanse the hose of the colema apparatus by running a germicidal solution through the bucket and tubing. Also, always keep a protective lid on the colema bucket to avoid the settlement of hair, dust, dirt, or other debris in the bucket. Always rinse the bucket thoroughly before and after using it.

Know Your Water

Not all household water is suitable for use in a colema. Don't assume that your water is safe for this use—or for drinking—if you have not had it tested or been assured in some way of its potability. Most local health departments offer a water-testing service to determine if water is safe to drink. However, it is my opinion that not all water deemed potable is adequate for use in a colema. Potability isn't the only consideration for persons who are concerned about chemicals in water. The chemicals often added to municipal water supplies to reduce bacterial counts, as well as other chemicals that may be present in water, may be undesirable for a colon cleansing. If your water has chemicals such as chlorine and fluoride, use an appropriate filtration process to remove them. Contact a water-conditioning company for help. As a last resort, you can purchase bottled water for use with your colema.

PROCEDURES IN THE SEVEN-DAY CLEANSING PROGRAM

In addition to the following procedures, you may wish to have massages, foot reflexology, or Epsom-salt baths during the Seven-Day Cleansing Program.

Starting the Cleanse

The evening before starting the cleansing program, take two herbal laxative tablets. To ensure a more thorough elimination, use an infant rectal syringe to inject one cup of olive oil into the rectum. Retain the oil until morning, if possible.

Skin Brushing

Your daily regimen should begin with skin brushing for a period of three to five minutes. I believe skin brushing is one of the finest of all "baths." No soap can wash the skin as clean as the new skin that you have under the old. You make a new top layer of skin every twenty-four hours. Skin brushing removes the old top layer and lets this clean new layer come to the surface.

The skin is one of the five main elimination channels of the body, throwing off about two pounds of toxic material each day in the form of perspiration. The skin has been called the third kidney because of its ability to rid the body of toxic waste material. Do not hinder the skin by using oils, cremes, or other noxious glop that serves only to clog it in the name of beauty. Instead, see what regular skin brushing can do for you.

Skin brushing is accomplished using a natural-bristle brush with a long handle to reach those hard-to-get-at places. The whole body (except the face) should be brushed one-half hour after rising and prior to the morning bath or shower. You may wish to skin brush again before retiring for the night. Note the powder that comes off your skin as you brush. These are crystals of uric acid and other dried waste products that came out with the perspiration.

Always brush the skin when it is dry, and never expose the brush to water. Although the bristles may seem a bit stiff at first, this is because the brush is new and your skin is not yet used to the brushing. If you find the brush is too stiff, you may, just once, hold the bristles in hot water for no longer than one minute and no deeper than one-half inch. This will soften the bristles a little. However, it will not be long before you desire a stiffer brush! Your skin will love you for brushing it regularly, and you will love the way your skin feels and looks, too.

Taking the Cleansing Drink

The Cleansing Drink should be taken five times daily. Take the first drink of the day at 7 A.M. Every three hours, on the hour, take another. The last drink of the day should be at 7 P.M.

The drink consists of two parts, which should be mixed separately and drunk in succession. The recipe is as follows:

Part One

8 ounces water
2 ounces apple juice
1 tablespoon clay water
1 rounded teaspoon intestinal cleanser

Part Two

10 ounces water
1 tablespoon apple cider vinegar
1 teaspoon raw honey.

1. Place the Part One ingredients in a 1-pint jar and screw the lid on tightly.

2. Place the Part Two ingredients in a large drinking glass.

3. Shake the Part One ingredients vigorously and drink the mixture immediately, since it will thicken to a gel-like consistency quite rapidly.

4. Immediately stir and drink the Part Two mixture. (The Part Two mixture, however, will not thicken like the Part One mixture, so you do not have to hurry as much.)

After taking the Cleansing Drink, wait at least fifteen to twenty minutes before getting on the colema board. Also wait at least fifteen to twenty minutes after finishing a colema to take a Cleansing Drink.

Taking the Supplements

The supplements should be taken four times each day, every three hours, beginning at 8:30 A.M. and concluding at 5:30 P.M. (For the exact schedule, see "Daily Schedule for the Seven-Day Cleanse" on page 130.)

It is easiest to lay out the whole day's supplements at the beginning of each day. Divide the supplements among four containers (small paper cups are handy for this), one for each interval. Different doses are required on days one, two, and three. Days three through seven require the same doses. Along with the pill supplements, you will be taking cod liver oil and liquid calcium-magnesium.

Eat no food other than the specified supplements and drinks for the full seven-day period. If you experience a feeling of extreme hunger, you may drink water, herbal tea, diluted fresh vegetable juice, clear vegetable broth, or Potato Peeling Broth (see below for a recipe). Plenty of liquid is essential to the success of the cleansing program. After taking the supplements, wait at least fifteen to twenty minutes before getting on the colema board. Also wait at least fifteen to twenty minutes after finishing a colema to take the supplements.

Taking the Flaxseed Tea

Flaxseed tea should be taken with the supplements at 8:30 A.M. and 5:30 P.M. To prepare the tea, use one rounded teaspoon of flaxseed in one and one-quarter cups of water for each cup of tea. Bring the mixture to a boil, then turn off the heat and let it sit until cooled. Store it in the refrigerator.

Flaxseed is available at most health-food stores. The tea it makes

Potato Peeling Broth

Potato Peeling Broth is an excellent source of organic potassium. It also tastes good.

2 to 3 medium-sized potatoes
3 cups water
1 celery stalk, chopped (optional)

1. Peel the potatoes, making the peelings about one-eighth to one-fourth inch thick.

2. Place the potato peelings and the water in a medium-sized saucepan. If desired, add the celery for additional flavor. Bring to a slow boil over medium heat, then reduce the heat and simmer until the peelings are soft, about fifteen minutes.

3. Using a slotted spoon, remove and discard the potato peelings and celery. Allow the broth to cool slightly.

4. Ladle the broth into a large mug and drink warm.

This recipe makes two servings. Store any remaining broth in the refrigerator. Warm the broth before drinking it.

is slippery and mucilaginous. If desired, strain the tea and discard the seeds.

Taking the Colema

The following detailed instructions explain the procedure and operation of the colema. (For quick instructions, see "The Colema, Step by Step," below.) I have endeavored to employ the most thorough, efficient, and natural means available to reach the goal of tissue detoxification and cleansing. The colema board was designed to provide a safe and easy way to take a high-colon cleanse. Once you are in the correct position, you can relax and virtually enjoy the rest of the procedure. Both your hands will be free, enabling you to massage your abdominal area, which is most important for optimum results.

The Colema, Step by Step

To ensure that your colema is safe and comfortable, simply follow these steps:

1. Lift the toilet seat and position the colema board so that it rests on the toilet with the splash shield above and around the opening. Support the other end of the colema board with a bucket, a stool, a chair, or the bathtub. The end on which your head will rest should be an inch or two higher.

2. Position the four- to five-gallon plastic bucket at least three to four feet above the board. The filled bucket can be hung if its weight can be supported safely. Be sure of the strength of your support.

3. Make sure the hose clamp is tight enough so that no water can pass it. Then start the siphon action by holding the end of the tube under a faucet and filling the tube with water. When the tube is full, place your finger over its end to prevent water loss and hang the plastic U-shaped tube over the bucket rim. Carefully let the end

you are holding fall into the bucket, which should be almost full of prepared colema water. The siphoning action will work when you release the clamp.

If you have installed a spigot in the bucket, simply remove the *U*-shaped tube, secure the hose clamp, and connect the longer segment of the hose directly to the spigot. Water will gravity-feed when the clamp is released.

4. Lubricate the rectal tip with K-Y jelly and insert the tip into the rubber connector tube.

5. Sit on the colema board facing the toilet. Draw your legs up so that your knees are bent and gently insert the lubricated rectal tip a maximum of three inches into your rectum. *Warning: Do not, under any circumstances, let the rectal tip enter your rectum more than three inches.*

6. Make yourself comfortable, with your knees bent and the soles of your feet resting on either side of the upright supports. Your buttocks should be in contact with these supports.

7. Once you are in a comfortable position with the rectal tip properly inserted, operate the hose clamp with your free hand, releasing the water solution. Continue until the bucket is empty, approximately one-half hour.

For a more detailed description of how to take a colema, see "Taking the Colema" on page 121.

Getting the Board Ready

First, lift the toilet seat. Now, place the working end of the colema board on the toilet. Support the other end of the colema board with a sturdy chair or stool, preferably just an inch or two higher than the toilet so that the board angles down to the toilet. You can see the correct setup in Figure 5.3. If you do not have access to a toilet, you can place an empty bucket under the working end of the board. In this case, you will need a container strong enough to bear your weight. If the bucket does not also function as the support, make sure that there

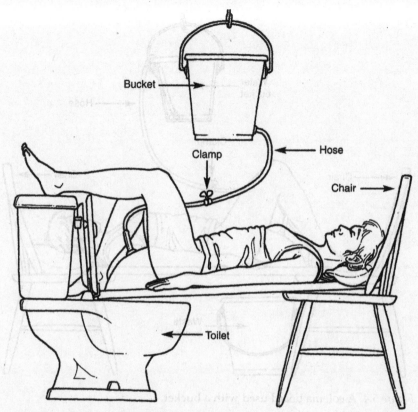

Figure 5.3. A colema board used with a toilet.

is minimal space between the top of the bucket and the underside of
the colema board to prevent splashing. A setup using a bucket can be
seen in Figure 5.4. If you desire, and there is enough room, you can
place the entire setup in a bathtub as a protection against spills.

Next, if you wish, you can place a folded towel on the board to
provide a cushion for your back. You can also place a comfortable pillow at the upper end of the board for your head. I like to use one of
those special pillow supports made for reading in bed.

Preparing the Water Bucket

Now it is time to prepare the water bucket. Place the water bucket on
a sturdy support from two to four feet above the colema board. Remember, five gallons of water weighs forty pounds! For this reason, it
is inadvisable to hang the bucket unless the bucket and handle are

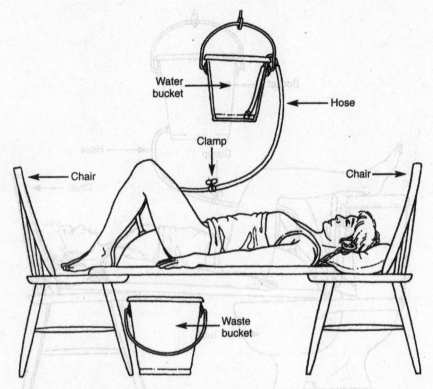

Figure 5.4. A colema board used with a bucket.

strong enough to support the weight. Fill the bucket almost to the top with body-temperature water. Be sure to leave room for any recommended additives you may want to put in the water. (See "Colema-Water Additives" on page 125.) You can place those additives in the water at this time.

Connecting the Apparatus

After you have prepared your colema water, attach one end of the hose supplied with your colema board to the bucket spigot or set up a siphon arrangement. (See "Siphoning the Colema Water" on page 127.) Make sure the shut-off clamp is in place, and attach the other end of the hose to the plastic elbow that passes through the splash shield. If you experience difficulty getting the rubber hose to slide over the fittings on either the bucket or the board, use a very small amount of K-Y jelly as a lubricant. Do *not* use petroleum jelly or a petroleum-based lubricant, as this can cause the rubber tubing to deteriorate.

Colema-Water Additives

Several ingredients can be added to the colema water for different purposes. The most popular and highly recommended are clay water, garlic, flaxseed tea, and liquid chlorophyll.

CLAY WATER

Clay water makes the colema an even more effective colon cleanser because it attracts a number of undesirable chemicals and removes them from the body. Use clay water only in your evening colema, however.

Add one-quarter to one-half cup of clay water to five gallons of colema water. Stir to mix.

GARLIC

If you think you may have worms or other intestinal parasites, garlic is an excellent colema additive. Even if you do not have intestinal parasites or are unsure, it is a good bowel cleanser. Do not mix garlic with clay water.

To prepare the garlic additive, place four clean and unpeeled garlic cloves in a blender with one cup of water. Liquefy the garlic. Strain and add the garlic water to the colema water.

FLAXSEED TEA

Flaxseed is also known as linseed because this small, brown, flat, football-shaped seed is high in linolenic acid, the most important of the essential fatty acids. When placed in water, brought to a boil, and allowed to steep, flaxseed releases a water-soluble mucilaginous gel with excellent lubricative properties that is very soothing to the digestive tract.

To make flaxseed tea, see the recipe on page 120. Use about one cup of strained tea in five gallons of colema water.

LIQUID CHLOROPHYLL

Very wonderful for the bowel, liquid chlorophyll is soothing and reduces swelling, inflammation, and pain. It cleanses, disinfects, and deodorizes, too. Liquid chlorophyll, in
fact, is the greatest natural cleanser and detoxifier known.
For these and other reasons, liquid chlorophyll adds to
the cleansing and restorative effectiveness of the colema
process.

To use liquid chlorophyll in the colema water, add one
teaspoon for every two quarts of water. Combining liquid
chlorophyll with flaxseed tea is especially effective.

Insert the colema tip far enough into the rubber tube that extends
from the splash shield so that no more than two and one-half to three
inches of the plastic rectal tip extend beyond the upright buttock supports. This is important. It serves as an additional precaution against
inserting more than three inches of the rectal tip into your rectum. If
you find that the rectal tip is too long, you will have to cut it down to
size. Most commercially supplied rectal tips do come longer than necessary. Presently, there are two types of rectal tips—a soft, anatomically curved type and a more rigid, straight type. Both are made of
plastic. The softer tip can be cut with a sharp knife or shears. The
more-rigid tip can be scored with a sharp knife and snapped in two.
*Warning: If you cut or snap the rectal tip, make sure you insert the uncut
end in your rectum.*

Inserting the Tip

Finally, apply a small amount of K-Y jelly to the end of the rectal tip
and insert the tip very carefully into your rectum to a maximum of
three inches. (See Figure 5.5.) Do this by slowly and carefully sliding
down the board until your buttocks come into contact with the upright supports, which are curved to permit a more or less watertight
seal. The rectal tip should enter the rectum easily and without discomfort. If you experience any discomfort in the rectum as you slide
down the board toward the buttock supports, stop immediately. Carefully withdraw the tip and check again to make sure the tip cannot
enter the rectum more than a maximum of three inches when the but-

Siphoning the Colema Water

If your bucket does not have a spigot or tap near the bottom, you have a situation in which the colema hose must be positioned over the rim of the bucket. You must siphon the water in order to get it to flow down to the colema board. Once the water has begun to flow, however, it will continue to flow until the bucket is empty or the water is turned off by squeezing the clamp.

Siphoning is accomplished by putting the end of the hose that goes in the bucket under a water faucet. Run water through it, past the plastic U-shaped tube, then hold it up in the air so that the water runs down into the long part of the hose. Once the water has run down, close the clamp, put the weighted portion of the tube back into the bucket, and hang the plastic U-shaped tube on the rim. You can then start the water flow by releasing the clamp. The idea here is that when water is pulled down the long part of the hose, it naturally draws the water from the bucket up the hose and around the U-shaped tube.

To retain the siphon potential, always clamp off the hose before the bucket runs dry. Clamping off the hose retains the pull of gravity without your having to repeat the start-up procedure. If the hose does run dry, you must repeat the siphon start-up procedure just described.

Another way of draining the bucket is to attach a small spigot at the base of the bucket. Attach the hose to this fitting, with the other end attached to the plastic tube at the business end of the colema board. Such a modification will render siphoning unnecessary. A spigot of the correct type and size is available in hardware stores.

tocks are in contact with the supports. This is most important. (For a further discussion of this, see "Insertion of the Rectal Tip" on page 129.)

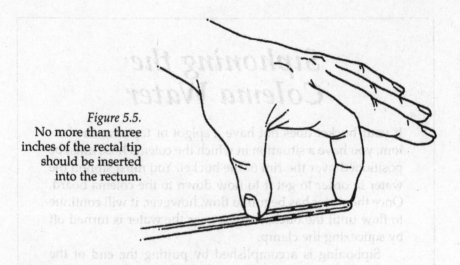

Figure 5.5.
No more than three
inches of the rectal tip
should be inserted
into the rectum.

Beginning the Cleansing Action

Once you are comfortable on the colema board, you can open the clamp to allow the colema water to flow into your colon. One of the major differences between the colema and the enema is that with the colema, the rectal tip is not removed until the cleanse is completed. The fecal matter will easily pass around the tip, allowing normal bowel action. The colema procedure encourages normal evacuation without producing bowel distention.

Massaging Your Abdomen

As you take the colema, massage your abdomen. A tennis ball is a most useful tool for this. Start massaging on your left side, rolling the ball with the palm of your hand while pressing it into your abdomen, but not so much that you make yourself uncomfortable. If you don't have a tennis ball, just keep your fingers together and use their flat surfaces to massage the abdomen. If you find any tender or sore areas, continue to massage until the tenderness is relieved. Continue up to your ribs on the left, then move across your abdomen and down the right side. This helps the water to get over and into the ascending colon.

If cramping occurs or the need to eliminate presents itself, simply relieve yourself as you normally would. The incoming water flow will temporarily halt from the pressure of the outgoing waste water and will automatically resume when you relax your abdominal muscles again. Continue in this manner until you wish to stop or the bucket is

Insertion of the Rectal Tip

It is very important that when you take a colema, you do not insert the rectal tip more than three inches past the anus.

The bowel bends at the sigmoid flexure, which is about four inches from the anus in the average person, perhaps less in some individuals. Inserting the tip more than three inches may bring excessive pressure to bear against the bowel wall at this bend, resulting in irritation, pain, and possibly mechanical problems. There should never be any force exerted on the bowel wall with the rectal tip.

To ensure your well-being, I recommend that you measure three inches from the end of the rectal tip and place an indelible mark there. Then, wrap a rubber band several times around the tip at the three-inch mark. Please note that I recommend using the soft-plastic rectal tip, which is flexible and will slide into the anus even in cases of hemorrhoids. Insert the tip to a maximum of three inches whether you use the soft or hard tip. Using the soft tip is an extra safety precaution, although I have experienced no problems with the hard type.

You must also be absolutely sure to insert the rectal tip by yourself. Never let another person insert it for you.

empty. It normally takes about thirty minutes to empty one bucket. If you are not finished eliminating and have exhausted the water supply, you can refill the bucket with enough water to finish. You may find it helpful to have someone ready to refill the bucket.

Completing the Colema

Upon completion of the colema, be very careful getting off the board, as any water present can make the board or floor slippery. As soon as you get off the board, disconnect the tubing and remove the board from the toilet. (You can stand the board on end in the bathtub.) In the reclining position, you were unable to completely eliminate all the water from the upper regions of the colon. When you stand up, gravity will cause any water and material to flow into the rectum, where it may cause a natural but immediate urge to defecate. At this time, you will want the toilet to be readily available, not covered by your colema board.

Now that you are finished, you must clean the board and tubes with a good germicidal solution, as explained on page 116. When removing the rectal tip for cleaning, be sure to replace the piece of quarter-inch tubing that holds the tip on the adjustable holder of the rectal tube. It is suggested that the tube be stored immersed in a germicidal solution such as Rugged Red until the next colema.

Now, doesn't it feel good knowing all that toxic material is gone?

DAILY SCHEDULE FOR THE SEVEN-DAY CLEANSE

The Seven-Day Cleansing Program will provide you with the opportunity to experience the benefits of a clean, efficiently working body. Many people report a sense of mental clarity and exhilaration that they never felt before. Let yourself relax and enjoy the following seven-day schedule:

Day One

7:00 A.M. Start the day with skin brushing. Follow with a Cleansing Drink and a shower.

8:30 A.M. Take the following supplements with flaxseed tea and 2 tablespoons (or the dose recommended on the bottle) of liquid calcium-magnesium:

- ❏ 12 tablets of chlorella *or* 8 tablets of alfalfa
- ❏ 1 tablet (or your preferred dose) of niacin
- ❏ 1 capsule of wheat germ oil
- ❏ 2 tablets of vitamin C
- ❏ 4 tablets of digestive-enzyme supplement
- ❏ 2 tablets of whole beet juice concentrate
- ❏ 1 tablet of dulse

10:00 A.M. Have a Cleansing Drink.

11:30 A.M. Take the same supplements as at 8:30 A.M., but this time with broth.

1:00 P.M. Have a Cleansing Drink.

2:30 P.M. Take the same supplements as at 8:30 A.M., but this time with herbal tea or broth.

4:00 P.M. Have a Cleansing Drink.

5:30 P.M. Take the same supplements as at 8:30 A.M., but this time with flaxseed tea.

7:00 P.M. Have a Cleansing Drink.

7:30 P.M. Take your first colema (with clay water added, if desired). Rest for one-half hour following the colema.

9:30 P.M. Take 2 tablespoons of liquid calcium-magnesium and 2 capsules of cod liver oil, then retire for the night. (Bedtime should be no later than 9:30 P.M.)

Day Two

7:00 A.M. Start the day with skin brushing. Follow with a Cleansing Drink.

7:30 A.M. Take a colema (with garlic, flaxseed tea, or liquid chlorophyll added, if desired). Rest for one-half hour following the colema, then take a shower.

8:30 A.M. Take the following supplements with flaxseed tea and 2 tablespoons of liquid calcium-magnesium:

❏ 18 tablets of chlorella *or* 8 tablets of alfalfa

❏ 1 teaspoon of liquid chlorophyll in a glass of water

❏ 2 tablets (or your preferred dose) of niacin

❏ 1 capsule of wheat germ oil

❏ 2 tablets of vitamin C

❏ 4 tablets of digestive-enzyme supplement

❏ 2 tablets of whole beet juice concentrate

❏ 1 tablet of dulse

10:00 A.M. Have a Cleansing Drink.

11:30 A.M. Take the same supplements as at 8:30 A.M., but this time with herbal tea or diluted juice.

1:00 P.M. Have a Cleansing Drink.

2:30 P.M. Take the same supplements as at 8:30 A.M., but this time with herbal tea.

4:00 P.M. Have a Cleansing Drink.

5:30 P.M. Take the same supplements as at 8:30 A.M., but this time with flaxseed tea.

7:00 P.M. Have a Cleansing Drink.

7:30 P.M. Take a colema (with clay water added, if desired). Rest for one-half hour following the colema.

9:30 P.M. Take 2 tablespoons of liquid calcium-magnesium and 2 capsules of cod liver oil, then retire for the night. (Bedtime should be no later than 9:30 P.M.)

Days Three Through Seven

7:00 A.M. Start the day with skin brushing. Follow with a Cleansing Drink.

7:30 A.M. Take a colema (with garlic, flaxseed tea, or liquid chlorophyll added, if desired). Rest for one-half hour following the colema, then take a shower.

8:30 A.M. Take the following supplements with flaxseed tea and 2 tablespoons of liquid calcium-magnesium:

    ❑ 18 tablets of chlorella or 8 tablets of alfalfa

    ❑ 1 teaspoon of liquid chlorophyll in a glass of water

    ❑ 3 to 4 tablets (or your preferred dose) of niacin

    ❑ 1 capsule of wheat germ oil

    ❑ 8 tablets of vitamin C

    ❑ 6 tablets of digestive-enzyme supplement

    ❑ 2 tablets of whole beet juice concentrate

    ❑ 1 tablet of dulse

10:00 A.M. Have a Cleansing Drink.

11:30 A.M. Take the same supplements as at 8:30 A.M., but this time with herbal tea or diluted juice.

1:00 P.M. Have a Cleansing Drink.

2:30 P.M. Take the same supplements as at 8:30 A.M., but this time with herbal tea.

4:00 P.M. Have a Cleansing Drink.

5:30 P.M. Take the same supplements as at 8:30 A.M., but this time with flaxseed tea.

7:00 P.M. Have a Cleansing Drink.

7:30 P.M. Take a colema (with clay water added, if desired). Rest for one-half hour following the colema.

9:30 P.M. Take 2 tablespoons of liquid calcium-magnesium and 2 capsules of cod liver oil, then retire for the night. (Bedtime should be no later than 9:30 P.M.)

CONCLUDING THE SEVEN-DAY CLEANSE

Under certain conditions, you may want to use rectal implants following the colema. Although there are various types of rectal implants such as suppositories, the ones we use are placed in an infant rectal syringe and squeezed into the rectum.

If you have colitis or rectal bleeding, use an implant consisting of one cup of flaxseed tea and one to two tablespoons of liquid chlorophyll. As an alternative, you can use three to five crushed chlorella tablets in one cup of water. To aid elimination, use one tablespoon of chlorella powder and one-half cup of clay water, adding enough distilled water to thin the mixture so that it will flow freely through the syringe.

Colemas are not habit-forming. In fact, I have found that colemas promote the restoration of natural regularity. Most of the people who complete the cleansing program return quickly to natural bowel movements. Regularity is best brought about through exercise, a proper diet and regular meal schedule, and the addition of fiber (from oat or wheat bran) to the diet. Make sure you get plenty of rest, and do not overwork yourself to the point of fatigue. In the unlikely event that you have trouble regaining normal bowel function following the cleanse, I recommend taking alfalfa tablets. These are high in fiber and contain chlorophyll. Fiber gives the bowel musculature something to "work against," and this provides a natural stimulation to the bowel. Chlorophyll is an excellent bowel cleanser. Take three to four tablets at each meal, making sure to chew or crack the tablets before swallowing them.

If you find that you have an excess amount of gas, your bowels do not move, or your anus is tense, you may be experiencing nervous strain. In this case, a glycerin suppository may help. Often, a warm cup of water infused into the rectum with an infant syringe will help the body relax enough to have a good bowel movement. Sometimes, drinking a glass of warm water will help. Unsalted sauerkraut is a good natural laxative that you can use at the first sign of constipation. It will not harm you in any way to continue using any of these methods until you once again have normal bowel movements. Never resort to unnatural chemical laxatives and risk the development of a bowel-debilitating laxative habit.

IN CONCLUSION

The Seven-Day Cleansing Program as presented here is often very helpful in relieving pain. Pain of all kinds from any part of the body— including joint pains associated with arthritis, and headache from migraine, tension, toxins, or another cause—will be relieved in the majority of cases. It should be understood that this treatment cannot be considered a cure-all, but rather an important step in leading the body to detoxification and cleansing. Serious medical problems should be referred to a physician.

You should follow the cleansing program at your own pace and watch for any reactions. Some people—especially the very toxic, the elderly, and the very weak—may have a negative response almost immediately. It may not be safe for you to stay on the program for more than one day if you experience a severe drop in your energy level or have another type of serious reaction.

This is the most powerful detoxifying program I know. Approach it with respect. You will be unleashing potent healing powers that may be overwhelming if you are uninitiated.

Although the Seven-Day Cleansing Program is a powerful detoxification procedure, I have found that most people with very chronic health problems cannot get rid of all the toxic material in a single cleanse. Additional cleanses are often necessary to bring about a thorough detoxification. You may need to repeat the seven-day cleanse a number of times in order to develop the necessary energy to eliminate more naturally and completely. You must remember that a tired and run-down body cannot eliminate as forcefully as it should. To restore the necessary energy to eliminate properly and to feel well takes time. Besides a cleansing phase, this program also has a phase in which building and restoration take place. Cleansing and building are partners with patience in the overall Ultimate Tissue Cleansing Program.

Chapter 6

The Seven-Week Building and Replacement Program

L ife in this world consists of an eternal cyclical pattern of building and tearing down, or positive and negative forces. The moon waxes and wanes, the tides ebb and flow, and the sun rises and sets. Everything in life needs to be periodically replaced or restored. If you own your own home, you know that worn or depleted things require restoration or replacement on a regular basis. Like all physical structures, the body requires a certain amount of care and maintenance to keep it functioning well and looking good. Part of that care is the nourishment that provides the materials to build cells, cells that eventually break down and need to be replaced by new ones.

We have just completed a cleansing, ridding the body of debris—worn-out cells, encrusted mucus, and other undesirable wastes. Although the Seven-Day Cleansing Program is a wonderful way to accomplish a major "housecleaning," it would be counterproductive and foolish to think we are finished now and do not need to worry about ongoing care. As good and beneficial as a cleanse may be, there is also a time for rebuilding. After cleansing, we must start replacement construction. After a period of restoration, we can cleanse again.

Many people think they can just keep cleansing without ever taking the time to restore and rebuild. Sometimes, people get too caught up in the spirit of cleansing and feel that they need to cleanse more and more. Unless we can achieve a balance between cleansing and restoration, we run the risk of becoming extremist. The seven-day cleanse, to begin with, might be considered a more or less extreme measure to accomplish detoxification. Sometimes, we must resort to extreme measures to reach a limited and well-defined goal. It would be dangerous to dwell there, however, so we need to move away from cleansing in order to achieve balance. Following the replacement and building program described in this chapter will bring the required balance to the overall program.

The Seven-Week Building and Replacement Program is designed to be followed after the Seven-Day Cleansing Program has been completed. You should stay on this replacement regimen for seven weeks, then repeat the cleansing. I have found that a cleansing-to-building ratio of one to seven (one week of cleansing to seven weeks of building) is the finest way to really "come clean" and reinvigorate the whole body. This cycle completely and thoroughly removes the toxic material from the bowel and helps create clean, healthy tissues. This cleanse-build cycle should be continued for six to eight months.

THE TRANSITION DIET

It is most unwise to immediately resume your regular diet following a fast. Although some nutrients are taken on the Seven-Day Cleansing Program, it is better to proceed slowly at first. In general, the more extended and severe a fast is, the longer it should be before a regular diet is resumed. You can suffer ill effects from breaking a fast with copious amounts of food, especially the wrong kinds of food.

To carefully reintroduce your bowel to regular meals, I suggest that you break your fast with the following transition diet. This diet will prepare your digestive organs for normal functioning and will make the changeover from the seven-day cleanse to regular meals very smooth.

The transition diet is very short—just two days long. The recommended meal plans are:

Day One

Breakfast: Lightly steamed shredded carrots.

Lunch: Large salad; yogurt, cottage cheese, or a nut-milk drink.

Dinner: Large salad; one steamed vegetable.

Day Two

Breakfast: Fresh fruit or rehydrated dried fruit; cereal or soft-boiled egg.

Lunch: Large salad; one steamed vegetable; yogurt, cottage cheese, or a nut-milk drink.

Dinner: Large salad; one steamed vegetable; a protein such as broiled or baked fish, or tofu.

Take your time eating, and chew well. If you find yourself thirsty between meals, have herbal tea or juice. On Day Two of the transition diet, try to have fresh fruit for breakfast. If fresh fruit is unavailable, see Appendix A for directions on rehydrating dried fruit. On the third day following the cleanse, resume your regular diet.

PROBIOTIC SUPPLEMENTATION

Probiotics are the friendly bacteria that reside in the gastrointestinal tract. They should not be confused with *antibiotics*, such as penicillin, which are medications intended to destroy infectious organisms that cause sickness. When ingested or injected, an antibiotic destroys the bad bacteria in the patient's system, thus helping the patient to recover. However, it also destroys the good bacteria, not only depriving the body of the good bacteria's benefits, but also opening up space for other, possibly damaging organisms to proliferate. Probiotics do not *destroy* anything. What they do is make the conditions in the bowel extremely inhospitable for bad bacteria, inhibiting the growth of the bad bacteria and making room for more good bacteria to grow. They "monitor and control the growth of potentially harmful microorganisms in your body," according to Natasha Trenev in her book *Probiotics.* They "also can help cancel out the effects of toxins and environmental pollutants that you can't avoid."

The advantages of using probiotic supplements on a regular basis should by now be obvious. It can therefore be argued that probiotics, though not a cure-all, should be used not only when diseases have already made inroads, but also as ongoing preventives. The three primary types of probiotics are *Lactobacillus acidophilus,* which guards the large intestine; *Lactobacillus bifidus,* also known as bifidobacterium, which protects the small intestine; and *Lactobacillus bulgaricus,* which travels through the entire digestive system and gives the other two a helping hand.

Lactobacillus acidophilus is the best-known probiotic. To be effective, however, it must contain at least 200 million organisms per cubic centimeter. Although the experience of clinicians has been that *Lactobacillus acidophilus* needs to be taken in large doses to work, there have been cases in which daily doses as small as four ounces have proven satisfactory when mixed with like amounts of supplemental lactase. In about 75 to 80 percent of cases of noncomplicated constipation, *Lactobacillus acidophilus* therapy has given uniformly good results.

Lactobacillus bifidus therapy has also been shown to be effective. Dr. Paul Gyorgy of the Institute of Nutrition Academy of Medical Sciences in Russia has determined that the main component of the normal human intestinal flora is bifidobacterium. Bifidobacterium has been shown to readily establish itself and predominate in the intestinal tract of breastfed newborns. Very encouraging research in both Russia and Germany has demonstrated the health-promoting qualities of *Lactobacillus bifidus* when it is well-established in the colon.

Lactobacillus acidophilus, *Lactobacillus bifidus*, and *Lactobacillus bulgaricus* are all available in supplemental form, while *Lactobacillus bulgaricus* is also available in yogurt made from live cultures. *Lactobacillus acidophilus* and *Lactobacillus bulgaricus* come in capsule, tablet, liquid, and powder form, and *Lactobacillus bulgaricus* comes in powder form. All are available from a number of manufacturers and can be purchased in most health-food stores. All should be used prior to the expiration date indicated on the container. After being opened, the culture should be kept tightly sealed and stored in the refrigerator. It should also be kept out of the light. The liquid form should always be refrigerated, even before being opened.

THE DAILY ROUTINE

The goal of the Seven-Week Building and Replacement Program is optimum building and replacement of tissues. To ensure meeting this goal, you should do the following on a daily basis:

❑ Skin brush for three to five minutes.

❑ Have one Cleansing Drink in the morning and one in the evening. (For the recipe, see page 118.)

❑ Take a lactobacillus supplement for one month to help restore the natural flora to the colon. Follow the directions on the label of the particular product you use.

❑ Take the following supplements three times a day, with meals:
  • 1 tablet of whole beet juice concentrate
  • 1 tablet of dulse
  • 2 tablets of digestive-enzyme supplement
  • 1 capsule of wheat germ oil

❑ Take the following supplements twice a day, in the morning and in the evening:
  • 2 tablets of vitamin C

- 2 tablets (or your preferred dose) of niacin
- 1 tablespoon of liquid calcium-magnesium

❑ Take 2 capsules of cod liver oil once a day, in the evening.

❑ Drink Revitalizing Broth or Vital Broth. (For the recipes, see "Broths," below.) These may be taken between meals, in mid-morning or mid-afternoon.

❑ Take time out to rest during the day. The best period is about midday, between noon and 3 P.M. It is also best to go to bed no later than 9:30 P.M.

Broths

The following broths are good to drink between meals in the morning or afternoon while on the building and replacement program.

REVITALIZING BROTH

1 pint water
3 cups chopped vegetables (use 5 or 6 different non-gas-producing vegetables such as beets, carrots, potato peelings, celery, parsley, okra, chayote pear, or any kind of squash)

1. Place the water and vegetables in a blender, cover, and liquefy at high speed.

2. Pour the liquid into a large saucepan and bring to a boil over medium heat. Reduce the heat to low and simmer for three to five minutes. Allow the broth to cool slightly.

3. Ladle the broth into a large mug and drink warm.

VITAL BROTH

2 quarts distilled water
½ teaspoon vegetable-broth powder
3 cups finely chopped celery stalks

2 cups finely chopped celery tops
2 cups finely chopped carrot tops
2 cups finely chopped beet tops
2 cups finely chopped (¼-inch-thick) potato peelings
1 garlic clove, finely chopped
1 carrot, chopped (optional)
1 onion, chopped (optional)

1. Place the water, vegetable-broth powder, celery stalks and tops, carrot tops, beet tops, potato peelings, and garlic in a large soup pot. If desired, add the carrot and onion for additional flavor. Slowly bring to a boil over high heat, then reduce the heat and simmer until the vegetables are soft, about twenty minutes.

2. Strain the broth and allow to cool slightly.

3. Ladle the broth into a large mug and drink warm.

In addition to the foregoing daily items, take colemas as needed to assure at least one bowel movement daily. Ideally, you should have two or three a day. Add flaxseed tea or clay water to the colema water, alternating them if desired. (For directions, see "Colema-Water Additives" on page 125.) I cannot make a generalization about how often to take a colema after the seven-day cleanse. Some people find colemas once a week to be ideal, while others need them more or less often. The important thing to remember is that you are striving for regular, easy bowel movements. If your health problems are difficult or have been chronic for a period of years, you probably will need to take a colema more often. If there is any question in your mind regarding your personal program, I recommend that you consult a nutritionist or holistic physician who understands natural healthcare. Always make sure that the things you do build a healthier body, and avoid falling into a situation in which you are merely treating a disease.

EXERCISE

In your ongoing care of the bowel and, for that matter, all the major elimination systems, you should not neglect exercise. When the muscles lack tone, prolapse of the abdominal organs is a possibility. The heart, lacking tone, cannot circulate the blood properly throughout the body. Likewise, the arteries and veins cannot contract enough to help the blood fight gravity and get to the brain tissues. The brain sends messages to the heart, and these messages are what keep the heart pumping. No organ can do without the brain.

Some people may have tried everything to get well, but still find their organs working under par. Many people do not realize that the energizing force for every organ in the body comes from the brain. Persons whose occupations require them to sit or stand continuously are less able to get blood to their brain tissues because their tired organs find it difficult to force the blood to ascend against the force of gravity. If we deny the brain tissues adequate blood, eventually every organ in the body will suffer.

One of the ways we can get better circulation to the brain and overcome gravity's effects on the internal organs including the bowel is the regular use of a slant board. When gravity exerts its force on the bowel, it pulls the bowel downward, which creates pressure on all the abdominal contents below the bowel. Exercising on a slant board is a good way to get the bowel back into its proper position. Exercises performed on a slant board are among the most helpful for the bowel and are absolutely necessary for regaining and maintaining good health.

In addition to helping the bowel, slant-board exercises are especially good in cases of inflammation and congestion above the shoulders, such as sinus trouble, bad eyes, falling hair, head eczema, ear conditions, and similar troubles. In many cases of heart trouble, fatigue, dizziness, poor memory, and paralysis, slant-board exercise helped more than any other treatment.

Slant-board exercises are basically the same all lying-down exercises. If you have a slant board that can be adjusted for height, you should set it so that the foot end is about eighteen inches off the floor. If you become dizzy when lying on the board, try setting the board a little lower. Some slant-board models are permanently fixed in height. If you become dizzy when first using a nonadjustable board, get off the board and lie on the floor until the dizziness passes. Then, try the slant board again. After one or two tries, you should not have any problem with dizziness.

At first, exercise for only five minutes a day on the slant board. As you get used to the board, you can gradually increase the time. The average person should lie on the board for ten minutes at 3 P.M. and again just before going to bed. Once you get into bed, lift your buttocks by positioning pillows under them to further help the organs return to a normal position.

A slant board should not be used by anyone who has uncontrolled high blood pressure, a heart condition, or cancer. It also should not be used by a pregnant woman or a woman experiencing a uterine hemorrhage.

The exercises shown in Figures 6.1 through 6.8 are especially good for prolapse of the colon and for regenerating the vital nerve centers of the brain. You can do one, two, or several of the exercises per session, and you can do them in any order you wish.

To perform the exercises shown in Figures 6.1 through 6.4, your feet must be secured by ankle straps. To perform the exercises shown in Figures 6.5 through 6.8, hold on to the handles of the slant board and remove your feet from the ankle straps. If your slant board is not equipped with handles, hold on to the sides of the board.

A wonderful slant-board exercise for the bowel is to lie down with your legs together and roll a tennis ball around your abdomen while applying pressure on the ball with the palm of your hand. The round surface of the ball will get right down into the bowel and exercise it.

SITZ BATHS

Sitz baths, particularly cold-water baths and hot-cold contrast baths, are an effective remedy for a sluggish bowel because they stimulate circulation in the pelvic area and increase nerve activity. To take a sitz bath, sit in a bathtub with the water rising only five inches up your body. Since only the pelvic region should be submerged in the water, sit with your feet on the rim of the tub or on top of something placed in the tub to prevent them from making contact with the water.

A sitz bath is best taken in the evening just before going to bed, but it can also be taken first thing in the morning. Although sitz baths can be taken with either hot or cold water, the most effective kind is the contrast bath, which employs both. First sit in cold water for one minute, then immediately switch to warm water for an additional few minutes.

Continue taking sitz baths for a period of three months. Sitz baths help not only bowel problems, but also many kinds of bladder and prostate problems.

THE HEALING CRISIS

If you diligently followed the tissue-cleansing program set forth in this book, are following a healthy diet, and continue to live a healthy

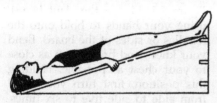

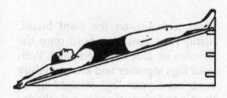

Figure 6.1. Lie on the slant board, your feet secured in the ankle straps. Rest your arms at your sides and relax, allowing gravity to help your abdominal organs back into their correct positions. For best results, lie on the board for at least ten minutes.

Figure 6.2. Lie on the slant board, your feet secured in the ankle straps. Stretch your arms over your head for a few seconds, then relax and return your arms to your sides. Repeat ten to fifteen times. This exercise stretches the abdominal muscles and pulls the abdominal organs toward the shoulders.

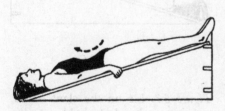

Figure 6.3. Lie on the slant board, your feet secured in the ankle straps and your arms at your sides. Inhale and, while holding your breath, contract your abdominal muscles to bring your abdominal organs toward your shoulders. Exhale and relax. Repeat ten to fifteen times.

Figure 6.4. Lie on the slant board, your feet secured in the ankle straps. Stretch your upper body to the right while vigorously patting the left side of your abdomen ten to fifteen times with both hands. Then, stretch your upper body to the left while vigorously patting the right side of your abdomen ten to fifteen times with both hands. Finally, raise your body to a sitting position and lower it back down again using your abdominal muscles. Repeat the entire sequence three to four times.

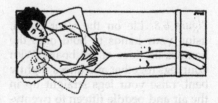

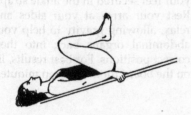

Figure 6.6. Lie on the slant board, using your hands to hold onto the handles or sides of the board. With your legs together and knees slightly bent, raise your legs straight up in the air and circle them in a clockwise direction eight to ten times. Repeat in the other direction. Lower your legs back onto the board and relax. Gradually increase the number of rotations in each direction to twenty-five over a two-week period.

Figure 6.5. Lie on the slant board, using your hands to hold onto the handles or sides of the board. Bend your knees and bring them as close to your chest as possible. Holding this position, first turn your head from side to side five to six times. Then, lift your head slightly and move your head and neck in a circular motion three to four times. Lower your head and legs back onto the board and relax.

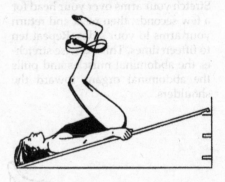

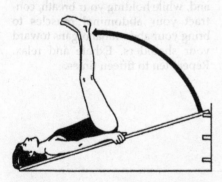

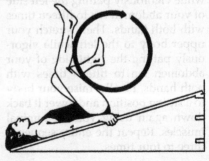

Figure 6.7. Lie on the slant board, using your hands to hold onto the handles or sides of the board. Slowly raise your legs straight up in the air, then slowly lower them back onto the board. Repeat three to four times.

Figure 6.8. Lie on the slant board, using your hands to hold onto the handles or sides of the board. With your legs together and knees slightly bent, raise your legs straight up in the air and peddle fifteen to twenty-five times as if you were riding a bicycle. Lower your legs back onto the board and relax.

lifestyle, you will at some time experience what is known as a healing crisis. A healing crisis is nothing to fear. On the contrary, this type of crisis is what you have been working for, and you ought to welcome it.

A healing crisis is a blessing in disguise. It is the result of an industrious effort by every organ in the body to eliminate waste products, and it sets the stage for the regeneration of weakened tissues. The healing crisis conforms with Hering's Law of Cure and is a natural result of it. Through a constructive and healthful process involving cleansing, good nutrition, and improved lifestyle, old tissues are replaced with new.

The healing crisis is called a crisis because it makes you feel as if your acute condition has returned. You experience the same symptoms you had when your condition was at its worst. In a disease crisis, you also experience these symptoms, but the symptoms are due to tissue breakdown and dysfunction, not renewed tissue activity and waste elimination.

Elimination is the most important difference between a healing crisis and a disease crisis. As part of its preparation for the healing crisis, the body eliminates toxic wastes including any chemicals and drugs. Drugs are suppressive and may cause iatrogenic disease (a condition brought on by a caretaker's diagnostic procedures or treatment), which only compounds the original problem. More frequently, they cause patients to suffer annoying new symptoms, so-called side effects. Physicians all too often then prescribe additional medications for the side effects.

Another sign of a healing crisis is that prior to and during the crisis, bowel elimination is very good. The bowel movements are natural and occur without difficulty. All the elimination organs do their part. In a disease crisis, elimination is usually not very good before the crisis and is unsatisfactory or stops completely during the crisis.

In a healing crisis, catarrh and waste that have been stored in the body are eliminated. The crisis is the final purifying process as the last of the waste is liquefied and thrown off. In a disease crisis, catarrh is not eliminated, and mucus is old, thick, chronic, and congestive.

Both healing crises and disease crises can come without warning. In general, you will know you are going through a healing crisis if you felt wonderful in the days prior to its onset. A healing crisis comes as an explosion, so to speak. It comes on suddenly, out of the blue, just as you're feeling your best. You will wonder how it could have come on so suddenly just when you seemed to have put your health problems behind you.

A healing crisis comes after the exchange of old tissue for new has been completed. It comes only when there is enough energy and activity available to the body as the result of the old, debilitated tissue being replaced with new. The old tissue has spent itself, and the new tissue, built from life-giving foods as well as through health-building processes, is strong and vital. When the body has regained its strength, it cleans house and violently throws off the old wastes in the form of a healing crisis.

To achieve regeneration of tissue, the body must pass through three stages. These three stages are the elimination, the transitional, and the building stages. The healing crisis usually occurs near the end of the transitional stage, which is when the new tissue has matured sufficiently to take on the function of a more perfect body.

Healing crises usually last about three days. They start with a slight discomfort, which quickly increases in severity until the point of complete expulsion is reached. During a healing crisis, a person may suffer old symptoms more severely than ever before. The person must "wait out" the crisis while continuing to follow a health-building path. Yielding to the temptation to resort to medications during this acute period will serve only to suppress the symptoms. The person will then have to again go through the crisis at a later time in order to be well.

Following the acute stage of the healing crisis, the discomfort diminishes. If the person's energy is low, the crisis sometimes lasts for a week or more. Healing crises affect patients with stronger vitality and greater energy more profoundly. Persons whose energy is too low do not have a healing crisis. Such persons must work to rebuild their health and energy until their bodies can manifest a crisis. Be assured that nature will not allow a healing crisis to take place before its appointed time.

HELPFUL HINTS FOR CONTINUED BOWEL CARE

Now that the Seven-Week Building and Replacement Program is behind you, you would be prudent to consider what you are going to do to maintain your good bowel function. A maintenance regimen should always include the following:

❑ Drink at least three glasses of liquid before having breakfast each morning. To maintain bowel regularity, it is often helpful to drink several glasses of water or a similar beverage before consuming your first meal of the day. Keep in mind that cold water will be delayed in the stomach, while warm water will pass directly to the bowel.

❏ Continue to take your probiotic supplements. Few people consume a diet that helps to maintain a natural balance of the colon bacteria. Earlier in this chapter I mentioned that lactobacillus supplementation should be continued for one month following the completion of the Seven-Day Cleansing Program. Some people, however, find that they need to continue bacterial supplementation indefinitely. Usually, this is because of a very chronic bowel condition or because the diet is not all that it should be. Through the use of technology, modern Americans have so adulterated their food that it no longer promotes friendly bacteria. Instead, it nourishes destructive bacteria. If we are going to live unnaturally, we would be wise to learn how to counteract some of the maladies that our style of living creates.

❏ Continue to take alfalfa tablets and digestive-enzyme supplements. I believe that both these supplements are very valuable items to take for an extended period while on the path to improved bowel and digestive health. You used both of these supplements on the Seven-Day Cleansing Program. As I mentioned in Chapter 5, alfalfa tablets often cause bowel gas, which is why I urged you to also take digestive-enzyme supplements. However, if you had a problem with bowel gas from the alfalfa tablets during the cleansing program, it by now may have already started to ease up or even have completely resolved. Nevertheless, I highly recommend that you continue to take the digestive-enzyme supplements.

❏ If desired, continue to use intestinal cleanser and clay water on a daily basis. Intestinal cleanser and clay water aid bowel elimination and regularity. For the intestinal cleanser, I recommend using one heaping teaspoon of psyllium-seed powder in eight ounces of water, mixing or shaking well. For the clay water, place one tablespoon of clay water in four ounces of water or add it to the psyllium-seed drink. If you wish, use clay water twice a day.

In addition to doing the foregoing items, there is also one thing that you should *not* do. Do not stop a discharge of any type. Always remember that old latent accumulations from the bowel turn into a catarrhal discharge as the body becomes strong enough to throw off these materials. These discharges will diminish and halt of their own accord as your body becomes clean on the inside. If you use medications to suppress a discharge, you may start yourself on the road to a growth or tumor. Therefore, never suppress a discharge. Let it flow, and continue with your health-building regimen until the discharge stops naturally.

PROPER FLORAL BALANCE

Our mode of living in this modern society tends to thwart any attempt to gain or maintain the proper intestinal flora, one of the requirements for a truly healthy gut. Intestinal flora, as discussed earlier in this chapter, are the microorganisms that live in the bowel. There is a great variety of these microscopic life forms, and they play a very important role in health and disease.

It is generally accepted that, in contrast to some animals, humans cannot digest cellulose (fiber) even though some of the bacteria present in the human digestive tract are capable of digesting minute amounts of this material. Other types of bacteria in the bowel play roles in the formation of vitamins B_1 (thiamine), B_2 (riboflavin), B_{12}, and K. The bacterial formation of vitamin K is especially important because food usually does not supply enough of this vitamin to maintain adequate coagulation of the blood. Other bacteria are beneficial because they help to keep the floral balance and thereby prevent various strains of coliform bacteria from overtaking the colon, which would cause fermentation and the formation of noxious bowel gas.

Where health and vitality are found, friendly and beneficial microbes invariably exist. Likewise, where decay and dysfunction are found, the microorganisms associated with disease are present. There is no aspect of earthly life in which some variety of bacteria does not play an important role. Bacteria are everywhere. We live in an ocean of them. All life on this planet is affected by their presence. The bacteria associated with disease, as well as those associated with health, work unceasingly via complex chemical reactions to bring about change.

The bacteria beneficial to humans hold the disease-producing organisms in check only if they are present in sufficient numbers. In the human colon alone, there are approximately four hundred to five hundred varieties of bacteria, fungi, yeast, and viruses. The specific varieties found in the center of the colon vary from those in the mucous lining, which are different from those that inhabit the right side of bowel, which are different from those that inhabit the left side of the bowel. Researchers have found evidence indicating that the mucus secreted by the intestine determines the kind of bacteria that will thrive there. In addition, they have found that it takes more than a year on average for a new diet alone to produce any noticeable change in the flora. Diet alone is too slow as a means of reinstating the necessary population of friendly bacteria.

When the body becomes polluted with toxic substances, the forces that maintain health and vitality diminish in proportion to the extent of the invasion. As they diminish, the disease-producing substances flourish. Such is the case with intestinal flora. Of all the things that alter the flora in the colon, medications are the most powerful. Broad-spectrum antibiotics are the worst of these offenders.

The word "antibiotic" is formed from the Greek words *anti*, meaning "against," and *bios*, meaning "life." Antibiotics are "against life." They are substances, natural or synthetic, that inhibit the growth of or destroy microorganisms. The killing-off of friendly bacteria by antibiotics can cause inflammation of the intestinal wall and overgrowth of yeast organisms. Antibiotics, as a rule, wreak havoc with the intestinal ecology and should, if at all possible, be avoided. An additional problem is that the overuse of antibiotics has led to the natural development of highly resistant strains of bacteria that can be combated only with ever-larger doses of antibiotics. In fact, some organisms have become totally resistant.

Many medications besides antibiotics also destroy friendly bacteria. The promiscuous use of over-the-counter nostrums such as antacids, pain killers, and other symptom-suppressing medications also has a detrimental effect on the lactobacillus bacteria in the bowel. When the floral balance in the intestinal tract is upset, it is very difficult for the person to return to optimal health. Bowel transit time, for instance, must return to normal, and bowel infections must be reduced.

In Chapter 3, I mentioned that the correct bacterial balance for a healthy bowel is about 85-percent friendly lactobacillus bacteria and 15-percent unfriendly bacteria such as *Bacillus coli*. In order to keep this balance, we must not do anything to destroy the friendly bacteria. We can build them up with food, of course, and with the proper nutrients, but this takes time. Some foods inhibit the friendly bacteria in the colon more than others. Cooked food, processed food, coffee, and alcohol all destroy friendly bacteria. The resulting floral imbalance makes it difficult to keep the bowel as clean as it should be. Long-term floral imbalance is a major reason so many people need bowel detoxification these days.

Ideally, we should never reach the point where our intestinal flora is unbalanced or we will need to go through a detoxification program. Parents should teach their children bowel hygiene when they are young. How to take care of the elimination system should be common knowledge and included in health or hygiene courses in school. The practices and processes that contribute to degeneration should be avoided, and persons who promote such abuses should be re-educated. Until our society realizes this, however, we must deal with the problem the best way we can, according to our individual beliefs.

COMPLICATIONS OF THE MODERN TOILET

No information on continued bowel care would be complete without mention of the device that we all must contend with—the modern toilet. It is my sincere belief that one of the bowel's greatest enemies in civilized society is the ergonomic nightmare known as the toilet or john. In "uncivilized" societies, people squat. In so doing, they avoid the complications associated with our "modern" plumbing fixture. In a natural squatting position, as seen in Figure 6.9, the bowel is supported and kept aligned by the thighs' contact with the abdominal wall, and many significant health benefits result. Figure 6.10 shows which sections of the bowel are supported by squatting.

We find that the American Indians never had any rectal problems or hemorrhoids. Why? They squatted to defecate. If you go to France, Italy, South America, or China, you will find that the toilet is often a hole in the floor and you have to squat to use it. As all of this shows, squatting is the normal eliminating position, the one in which all of the internal organs are held in proper position. When squatting is habitually used for elimination, no hemorrhoidal veins protrude from the rectum.

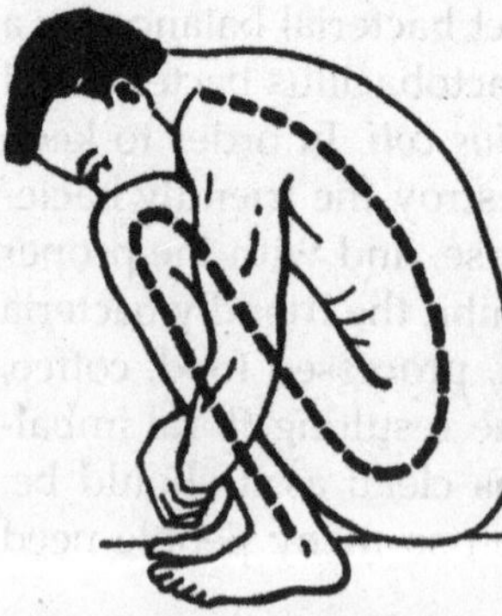

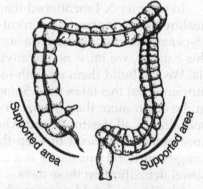

Figure 6.9. The natural squatting position.

Figure 6.10. The sections of the bowel that are supported by the thighs when a person squats.

The toilet first became popular in England in approximately 1850, and its use soon spread throughout the civilized world. It spread quickly because it came on the scene at the same time as plumbing, which allowed for the clean disposal of what previously was stored in chamber pots or dumped into the street. The toilet was originally designed by Alexander Cumming, a watchmaker, and was subsequently improved upon by Joseph Bramah, a cabinet-maker. These were not men of medicine, nor were they cognizant of human biomechanics, so they did not recognize the mechanical advantage that squatting offers the body. Likewise, the general public was unaware of the advantage, and therefore, the "new and improved" toilet quickly became established.

It was not until the early 1900s that certain doctors, faced with a dramatic increase in the incidence of bacterial disease, questioned the conventions of the time, the most suspect of which was the toilet. In *The Culture of the Abdomen*, written in 1924, the author quotes some of the leading medical authorities of the time, who were very outspoken about the toilet's faulty design and the ensuing health consequences. He stated, "It would have been better that the contraption had killed its inventor before he launched it under humanity's buttocks."

It is interesting to note that Dr. Denis Burkitt, the same medical doctor whose research verified the importance of dietary fiber (see page 52), also made observations about the squatting posture when he was attempting to learn why traditional African societies have little or no bowel cancer. Perhaps for the same reasons it took decades to disseminate his discoveries on the importance of dietary fiber, his observations on the posture of elimination were never publicized.

Constipation, hernias, varicose veins, hemorrhoids, and appendicitis have all been attributed to the use of the toilet. A solution to the dilemma was offered several years ago in the form of a footstool, used to elevate the feet while one is seated on the toilet, thereby approximating the squatting posture. This footstool was so popular for a while that it was sold at Harrods of London. To purchase the footstool in the United States, see Appendix B.

All of the undesirable consequences of using the toilet result from the simple action of sitting while bearing down, which robs us of the support to the abdominal wall and colon normally afforded by squatting. Figure 6.11 shows the posture normally held when sitting on a toilet, and Figure 6.12 shows the portions of the bowel that are compromised because of it.

The majority of all bowel problems are located in just two areas of the bowel—the cecum, in the lower right quadrant, and the sigmoid,

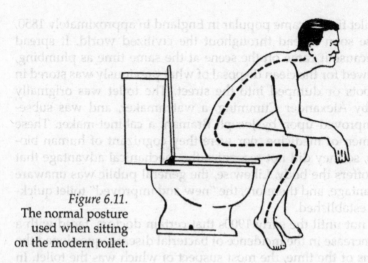

Figure 6.11.
The normal posture
used when sitting
on the modern toilet.

in the lower left quadrant. These two portions of the colon are the
very ones that are normally in contact with the thighs during squatting. When we use the toilet, we apply no mechanical pressure to
these areas, which allows fecal matter to stagnate there. As we have
seen, bowel-stagnation problems that result in poor elimination place
an additional toxic burden on the bloodstream and assert a negative
reflex effect on corresponding parts of the anatomy.

CONDITIONS ASSOCIATED WITH THE MODERN TOILET

A number of specific conditions are associated with the use of the
modern toilet. They include ileocecal-valve dysfunction, incomplete
elimination, and strictures in the sigmoid.

Ileocecal-Valve Dysfunction

When we bear down without the thighs physically supporting the
ileocecal valve, we compromise the valve's mechanical dynamics. The
valve is "blown out" and thus becomes unable to perform its function
of preventing the reflux of fecal matter into the small intestine. As a
result, fecal bacteria proliferate and travel up the small intestine, and
fecal toxins are absorbed into the bloodstream. These toxins dramatically increase the burden on the bloodstream, which negatively affects
all the other organs.

To add to the problem, gas or hard stool may form and cause pressure against the rectum. This problem is aggravated by the effects of

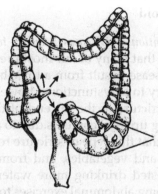

Figure 6.12. The sections of the bowel that are compromised by the lack of support afforded by the posture used on the modern toilet.

Unsupported areas

fatigue and the pull of gravity on the bowel. Fatigue results in loss of muscle tone in the bowel wall, while gravity encourages prolapse of the transverse colon.

When sitting on the toilet and bearing down, you exert force against the rectal tissues. To prevent this, keep your hands above your head when bearing down. In the bathrooms in my sanitariums, I have had a little rope installed above and to the side of each toilet. Holding onto such a rope when having a bowel movement effectively keeps the hands above the head.

The phenomenon of fecal bacteria and other fecal matter re-entering the small intestine is so common that the ileocecal valve is now being described in some medical textbooks as inherently incompetent. This viewpoint, however, stands in direct opposition to what was believed by anatomists and physicians of the past.

The major symptoms of ileocecal-valve dysfunction are low-back and hip problems, caused by the weakening of the muscles in the lower-right quadrant of the abdomen. Varying consistency of the stool with a tendency toward diarrhea and dark circles under the eyes are also symptoms of a dysfunctional ileocecal valve.

Incomplete Elimination

Dr. John Chiene clinically verified the incomplete elimination that people experience when using the toilet. He became so convinced that the toilet was faulty in design that he actually weighed and compared the fecal mass he passed using the toilet with what he passed in a squatting position. Based on his finding that he always eliminated less mass when using the toilet, he concluded that users of the toilet suffer from incomplete elimination.

Strictures in the Sigmoid

In his book *The Prevention of Diseases Peculiar to Civilization*, Sir W. Arbuthnot Lane stated that many of our most pressing concerns, such as cancer and heart disease, result from a toxic burden on the bloodstream that is secondary to a dysfunctional bowel. Dr. Lane eventually discovered that a stricture in the far end of the bowel acts like a plug in a drain, backing up fecal contents due to an incompetent ileocecal valve. He stated that this type of stricture results from an inadequate intake of fruits and vegetables, and from restraining normal elimination. He suggested drinking more water, eating fresh fruits and vegetables, and doing abdominal exercises to encourage the body to again have a bowel movement after every meal, "by which alone health, happiness and freedom from disease can be assured," he said. This standard for bowel function was originated by Hippocrates, the father of medicine.

Research by William Welles, D.C., a colleague and friend as well as a contributor to this book, indicates that strictures may result from tightening due to weakness created by a malfunctioning ileocecal valve. Dr. Welles was very heartened to learn that Dr. Lane was so concerned about the posture of elimination that he attempted to redesign the toilet. Both Dr. Welles and I believe that it is very important to educate our children and future generations about the health hazards of the toilet. It's time to break the short-lived and ignorant tradition of using the toilet by returning to the squatting posture. By adopting the squatting posture instead of sitting, we allow the bowel to resume its function as nature intended.

IN CONCLUSION

In the field of medicine, much time and money are spent patching up the effects of an environment that is actually toxic and hazardous to health. Most of today's doctors treat people for ailments that are the direct results of "civilized" living. These doctors don't focus on eliminating the causes of the disturbances. Instead, they treat the symptoms and leave their patients to continue to ignorantly and almost addictively tear themselves down. Lasting and abiding health is the result of education and discipline in cleanliness of the body, mind, and spirit. All else is a compromise at best.

Chapter 7

Nutritional Sins and Dietary Laws

To disobey the basic laws of the universe that govern our lives is to hasten our demise. To be sure, few people in today's modern society can live in complete accordance with the dietary laws, even if they so desire. Natural, pure, and whole foods are not always available. Our lives at the dawn of the twenty-first century often do not allow the simple living that is most conducive to mental and physical well-being. We can, however, make a reasonable attempt to do better than we have been doing. Avoiding a few simple things and doing a few others will go a long way toward ensuring a cleaner, better-functioning body. If we neglect to do these things, we commit nutritional "sins," which cause sickness and ill-health.

Nutrition and cleansing constantly interact and complement one another in normal body functioning. We have seen that the other side of cleansing is building and restoration. We restore and build with nutrition. Nutrition is the master science by which we supply the body with those elements essential to the building and maintenance of cellular structure and function. Structure is intimately related to function. It is a common saying in pathology that "disease is function gone wrong."

THE SIX NUTRITIONAL SINS OF CIVILIZATION

Human beings instinctively are evolving beings, seekers. They want to know what is on the other side of the fence. They want to improve their appearance. They want to eat, drive, and own the best. They understand, to one degree or another, that they can have what they want if they make the effort physically, mentally, and spiritually. However, I have found in my seventy years of practice that human beings can destroy their ability to attain their goals by committing the six nutritional sins and destroying their health.

My mother used to say, "Health isn't everything in life, but without health, everything else is nothing." People cannot reach their goals or live in happiness when their health is gone. The six nutritional sins are the causes of more health breakdowns than most people can imagine. No matter what a person's profession or daily routine, he or she causes problems in every organ and bodily function through the inadequate consumption of fiber; the consumption of too much fat and the wrong kinds of fats and oils; and the excessive consumption of pasteurized, homogenized dairy products, inorganic salt, sugar, and wheat.

The Inadequate Consumption of Fiber

Over the past few years, there has been a "bran craze" in the United States. Adding extra bran to the diet is necessary because our nutritional habits do not allow us to keep our bowels in good working order. Furthermore, some people look to oat bran as the means to lowering an excessive cholesterol level. Actually, eating bran does not have a direct effect on the cholesterol level. By decreasing the transit time of waste material through the bowel, fiber such as bran reduces toxic-waste buildup in the body. Researchers now think that fiber helps dietary cholesterol to be carried more rapidly through the bowel, thus reducing the chance of its being absorbed. It is interesting that in recent years the FDA has allowed food manufacturers to cite research on high-fiber diets when touting the health value of certain high-fiber breakfast cereals.

Although high-fiber diets are desirable, cholesterol can be lowered by more-efficient methods. Bran adds very little nutritive substance to the diet. Rather, its coarse protective covering acts as roughage, which naturally stimulates the bowel to move its contents along more quickly. This is the main function of bran. But fiber can also be found in foods that have a high mineral content such as fruits, vegetables, and whole grains.

Our ancestors didn't need to add bran to their diets. The eating habits of Americans have changed drastically since 1900. We eat less than two-thirds of the fresh fruits, vegetables, and grains that our grandparents did. At the same time, our diets consist of more refined and manhandled foods such as white flour and sugar products, as well as commercially packaged and preserved foods. Just as the quantity of high-fiber foods is considerably less than it was at the turn of the twentieth century, the quality of these foods is also greatly reduced. It is no wonder that we now have a higher percentage and earlier appearance of diseases such as diverticulitis, constipation, and colon cancer.

The average Western diet includes 11.0 grams of fiber, as compared to 24.8 grams of fiber in the diet of Bantu tribesman. In rural eastern Africa and other primitive societies, there is virtually no incidence of diverticulitis or colon cancer, unless the natives adopt a modern "civilized" diet, as they do when they move to urban areas. The research of British surgeon Denis Burkitt (see page 52) comparing the diets, bowel habits, and bowel-related diseases of rural eastern African natives with those of British citizens living in eastern Africa has shown that the high fiber content of the food used by the rural natives is the primary causal factor in the low incidence of bowel diseases among them. One of the main differences between the African natives and the British, whose diet is much lower in fiber than that of the natives, is that the British have a much slower bowel transit time and a significantly higher incidence of bowel diseases than the African natives.

Nowadays, the National Cancer Institute recommends a diet that supplies 20 to 30 grams of fiber per day. Even the American Cancer Society is now concerned with diet. Table 7.1 will give you an idea of how many grams of fiber are found in some common foods. Note that the figures supplied in the table are based on several sources that differ widely in the fiber contents they give for the foods listed. This table is provided only to give you a *general* idea of the fiber content of foods.

Table 7.1. Fiber Content of Some Common Foods

FOOD	AMOUNT	GRAMS OF DIETARY FIBER
Fruits		
Apple, unpeeled	1 medium	3.5
Banana	1 medium	2.4
Cantaloupe	¼ melon	1.0
Cherries, sweet	10 cherries	1.2
Orange	1 medium	2.6
Peach, unpeeled	1 peach	1.9
Pear, unpeeled	½ large	3.1

Table 7.1 (cont'd)

FOOD	AMOUNT	GRAMS OF DIETARY FIBER
Fruits (continued)		
Prunes	3 prunes	3.0
Raisins	¼ cup	3.1
Raspberries	½ cup	3.1
Strawberries	1 cup	3.0
Vegetables, Cooked		
Asparagus, cut	½ cup	1.0
Broccoli	½ cup	2.2
Brussels sprouts	½ cup	2.3
Parsnips	½ cup	2.7
Potato, unpeeled	1 medium	2.5
Spinach	½ cup	2.1
String beans	½ cup	1.6
Sweet potato	½ medium	1.7
Turnip	½ cup	1.6
Zucchini	½ cup	1.8
Vegetables, Raw		
Celery, diced	½ cup	1.1
Cucumber	½ cup	0.4
Lettuce, sliced	1 cup	0.9
Mushrooms, sliced	½ cup	0.9
Spinach	1 cup	1.2
Tomato	1 medium	1.5
Legumes		
Baked beans	½ cup	8.8
Kidney beans, cooked	½ cup	7.3
Lentils, cooked	½ cup	3.7
Lima beans, cooked	½ cup	4.5
Navy beans, cooked	½ cup	6.0
Peanuts	10 nuts	1.4
Peas, dried, cooked	½ cup	4.7
Breads, Pastas, and Flours		
Bagel	1 bagel	0.6
Bran muffin	1 muffin	2.5
French bread	1 slice	0.7
Oatmeal bread	1 slice	0.5

Pumpernickel bread	1 slice	1.0
Rice, brown, cooked	½ cup	1.0
Spaghetti, cooked	½ cup	1.1
Whole wheat bread	1 slice	1.4

Nuts and Seeds		
Almonds	10 nuts	1.1
Filberts	10 nuts	0.8
Popcorn, popped	1 cup	1.0

Breakfast Cereals		
All-Bran	⅓ cup	8.5
Bran Buds	⅓ cup	7.9
Bran Chex	⅔ cup	4.6
Corn Chex	⅔ cup	5.4
Cornflakes	1¼ cups	0.3
40% Bran–type	¾ cup	4.0
Oatmeal, regular, quick, or instant	¾ cup	1.6
Raisin Bran–type	¾ cup	4.0
Shredded Wheat	⅔ cup	2.6

E. Lanza and R.R. Butron: "A Critical Review of Food Fiber Analysis and Data." © 1986 The American Dietetic Association. Reprinted by permission from the *Journal of the American Dietetic Association*, Volume 86 (1986), page 732.

The Consumption of Too Much Fat and the Wrong Kinds of Fats and Oils

Surprisingly, fats are among the most useful foods, but they are also the most abused. Good fats and oils are efficient sources of energy, carry the fat-soluble vitamins to the cells, are necessary in the production of certain hormones, and make up the myelin sheath that covers and protects many of the nerve cells in the body and brain. The problem is too much fat and the wrong kinds of fats and oils. The average American diet is about 50-percent fats, mostly saturated fats, the animal fats that harden at room temperature. These fats are blamed for the high incidence of heart disease and other health problems.

Excess fat in the diet causes hardships for the liver and gallbladder, which aid in the digestion of fat. Heated fats and oils are among the biggest contributors to excess cholesterol formation in the body. We must stop taxing our bodies with pasteurized butters, roasted nuts, deep-fried foods, and other heated oils. Fatty foods such as

bacon, sausage, hamburgers, and foods fried in grease produce too
much cholesterol in the body.

Heated oils such as butter, margarine, and vegetable oils are
found in foods like cheeses and baked goods. In advertisements, the
manufacturers of children's snacks highlight the good ingredients—
for example, "real" fruit, granola, oats, yogurt, vitamins, and skim
milk—but neglect to mention the hydrogenated or partially saturated
vegetable oils and lard, sugars, and salt. Coconut and palm oil
account for most of the saturated fats found in pudding snacks and
"health" bars. These oils are saturated fats, which may not be harmful in moderate quantities—as long as they are not heated to high
temperatures.

Among the worst fats are the so-called partially hydrogenated
fats, which are artificially created. Oils—that is, fats that are naturally
liquid at room temperature—are hydrogenated to give them a creamy
consistency. Margarine is a prime example. These fats and oils are
dangerous because the hydrogenation process creates chemical compounds that do not occur naturally in foods. These chemical compounds' long-term effects on the body are not known. Always read
the label before buying any food product. You don't want anything
that contains partially hydrogenated ingredients. Food products that
contain these ingredients are what I call "manhandled foods." They
are created only for convenience and profit, and ignore your good
health.

Foods that supply good fats and oils include avocado, raw nuts,
fish, goat's milk, and seeds such as flaxseed.

The Excessive Consumption of Pasteurized, Homogenized Dairy Products

The dairy industry constantly promotes the notion that pasteurized
and homogenized milk is "good food," especially for children. Milk
products including cheese, buttermilk, ice cream, whey products, yogurt,
sour milk, cream products, and cottage cheese—all pasteurized and
some homogenized as well—account for 25 percent of the American
diet. I believe that 6-percent dairy products in a diet is sufficient.

The average daily food regimen is 54-percent milk and wheat. Are
we not ignoring the principle of variety? God's garden gives us a
healthy range of foods! Asparagus, beets, turnips, carrots, fruits,
berries, nuts, and all the other natural foods enable mankind to eat a
balanced diet. It is not natural, however, to have so much milk and
wheat in the diet.

Cow's milk and wheat are two of the greatest catarrh-producing foods. They are common allergens and often provoke an immune-system response, the result of which is a catarrhal condition. In moderate amounts, pasteurized milk and wheat are usually tolerated well. However, the American diet is overburdened with wheat and dairy, and this is one reason why people who consume such heavy amounts of these foods are overburdened with catarrh.

Not only is cow's milk catarrh-producing, but milk products today lack the quality they once had. Cows are not fed nutritionally balanced diets because farmers are paid for the quantity of milk they supply, not for the quality. Soil and fodder are often sprayed with chemicals that show up in the milk in the form of residues and eventually lead to allergies in many of the people who consume milk products.

Pasteurization may have been justified when milk-borne diseases such as bovine tuberculosis, transmitted from infected cows and associated with unsanitary milking conditions, were a threat to human health. However, pasteurization also kills important enzymes and reduces the nutritional value of milk. Raw milk contains phosphatase, an enzyme that is essential for calcium absorption. Although pasteurization does not deplete calcium, it hinders calcium absorption because it destroys the phosphatase enzyme.

With the cleanliness and health standards imposed on dairy farms today, pasteurization is hardly necessary. The FDA admits to this by certifying the farms that adequately meet its strict cleanliness requirements to sell raw milk. In other words, pasteurization is a way of letting farms get by with reduced standards of cleanliness. The name of the game here is money, not what is best for health. It costs more, and thus would increase milk prices, if more stringent cleanliness requirements were imposed on dairy farms.

Scientific research indicates that *homogenized* milk may be one of the contributing factors to atherosclerosis. According to Nicholas Sampsidis in his book *Homogenized!* milk fat contains an enzyme called xanthine oxidase. When milk is not homogenized, its fat and xanthine oxidase are digested in the stomach and small intestine. When milk is homogenized, its xanthine oxidase is not broken down, but instead passes into the circulation, where it damages arterial walls and heart muscle. Scar tissue and a buildup of calcified plaque on the arterial walls are the normal responses to this tissue damage. Cholesterol and fatty deposits are then laid down along the roughened surfaces of the scars and plaque, narrowing the passageway and obstructing the flow of blood.

It has been demonstrated in guinea pigs that pasteurization and heating of milk and other dairy products can contribute to conditions such as joint stiffness. Guinea pigs fed pasteurized skim milk developed joint stiffness, hardening of the arteries, and calcification of the soft tissues. When raw cream was added to their diet, these conditions were reversed. A factor in the cream of raw milk, the Wulzen factor, was credited with the reversal.

Probably the most famous experiments pointing out the difference between raw and pasteurized milk were conducted by Francis M. Pottenger, Jr., M.D., and clearly set forth in his book *Pottenger's Cats*. (See "Francis Marion Pottenger, Jr., M.D." on page 163.) A group of cats was restricted to a diet of raw milk and raw meat, while a second group was fed only pasteurized milk and cooked meat. By the second generation, the cats fed the pasteurized milk and cooked meat were unable to reproduce, while the other group remained healthy and normal. This classic experiment pointed out the benefits of raw foods as opposed to heated or cooked foods.

As I already mentioned, both pasteurization and homogenization are economically motivated. Pasteurization increases the shelf life of milk. In recent years, we have seen ultra-pasteurization (pasteurization at higher than normal temperatures) extend shelf life even longer. Homogenization forces people to purchase cream and milk separately, rather than to buy one bottle and pour the cream off the top, as used to be done. Pasteurization and homogenization serve merely as conveniences to increase profits for the dairy industry.

I recommend goat's milk, soymilk, and nut-milk drinks as substitutes for cow's milk. They do not produce problematic amounts of catarrh in the body. My recommendations are shared by many allergy specialists, whose first advice to their asthmatic patients is often to eliminate wheat and cow's milk from the diet. These simple changes often regulate these patients' allergies. Catarrh overloads the five main elimination channels of the body. When the elimination systems are overburdened, the result is a buildup of toxic material, which is at the root of many of today's health problems.

The Excessive Consumption of Inorganic Salt

When most of us think of salt, we think of common table salt. Table salt, or sodium chloride, is usually mined or obtained from evaporating sea water or Celtic salt. Our bodies require the chemical elements that salt provides. When salt is dissolved, its elements—sodium and chloride—are ionized and become two of the more important elec-

Francis Marion Pottenger, Jr., M.D.

Francis M. Pottenger, Jr., was the first-born son of Francis M. Pottenger, Sr., and Adelaide Gertrude (Kitty) Babbit. Francis, Sr., was the founder and operator of the internationally famous Pottenger Sanitarium and Clinic for Diseases of the Chest, located in Monrovia, California. The sanitarium, which operated from 1903 to 1956, specialized in the treatment of tuberculosis. Food was grown right on the sanitarium's farms, and the young Francis was exposed to the benefits of natural foods and what they could do for those in ill-health.

Francis, Jr., was very interested in mechanical things and possessed great inventive talent and an inclination towards engineering. His father, however, had other ideas for his son and insisted he become a physician. Accordingly, Francis entered his father's alma mater, Otterbein College in Westerville, Ohio, in 1921. He was an excellent student, and in 1930, he received his medical degree and began an internship at Los Angeles County Hospital.

While attending medical school, Francis, Jr., developed a disdain for the way modern civilized people treated themselves. He strove to understand how mankind could achieve better health and eliminate chronic illness. His quest led him back to his father's sanitarium, and between 1932 and 1942, he conducted feeding experiments to determine the effects of heat-processed food on cats. This was to become one of the most famous studies in nutrition. Dr. Pottenger determined that much chronic disease was caused by the failure to supply adequate nutrition through the intake of raw, uncooked, and unprocessed foods. He found that a diet of cooked, processed foods was detrimental to health. The complete and fascinating story of his experiment can be found in his book *Pottenger's Cats*.

trolytes present in our tissues. Due to their positive or negative charges, electrolytes are able to transfer electrical energy within the body. They also repel elements with like charges and attract those with opposite charges to form chemical bonds. Because of these actions, they are able to carry certain chemicals across cell membranes and to perform various other electro-chemical functions that are necessary to the well-being of the body.

We replenish our electrolytes from the foods we eat and the liquids we drink. Foods from plants and animals, especially fruits, are rich in electrolytes. Unlike table salt, which is obtained from nonliving sources, living (organic, biochemical) matter contains salts of a different nature. Organic foods—as opposed to manmade "foods" concocted from chemicals in a laboratory or "foods" from other inorganic sources—act differently in the body. The body, in its infinite wisdom, somehow knows the difference between organic and inorganic substances.

There is widespread misunderstanding of the words "organic" and "inorganic." "Organic" refers to anything pertaining to or derived from a living organism. "Inorganic" things do not involve either life processes or the products of life processes. Table salt is not, by this definition an organic substance.

(Keep in mind, however, that the preceding definitions of "organic" and "inorganic" should not be confused with the terms "organic" and "inorganic" as used in relation to the method of growing a food. Foods are "organically grown" when the plant as well as the soil in which the plant grew were free of chemical fertilizers, sprays, and insecticides. In other words, organic foods may or may not be organically grown. Inorganic foods, of course, can never be organically grown, since they are not grown.)

Many processed and packaged foods contain inorganic sodium in the form of additives such as preservatives or taste-enhancers. This sodium, like table salt, does not react in the body the same way the biochemical sodium contained in living foods does. Some scientists refute this notion. They claim that an element is the same whether it comes from an organic or inorganic source and that there is no difference in its action in the body. However, clinical experience does not show this to be the case. Salt, in fact, is a perfect example. Too much inorganic sodium, like that contained in table salt, increases the risk of hardening of the arteries, with its attendant elevations in blood pressure, increased risk of stroke, and other complications in certain people. Therefore, in recent years, medical nutritionists have advised against using too much table salt. In fact, many patients are now placed on strict salt-free diets to prevent further deterioration of their severely compromised cardiovascular systems.

Salt restriction is a mixed blessing, however, because, although it cuts down on the intake of inorganic sodium, it does nothing to supply the body with the necessary sodium from organic sources. Organic sources of sodium are also to be avoided on a salt-free diet. But foods naturally high in organic sodium pose no threat to health. This is because the sodium in organic foods is accompanied by other minerals and nutrients that slowly trickle into the cirulatory system and thus allow the bodily fluids to adjust and to provide the cells with the right amounts of potassium, magnesium, and calcium needed for bodily functions. Refined sodium chloride taken in high amounts floods the gastrointestinal tract, blood, lymph, and tissues with an excess of two highly reactive chemical ions, isolated from the substances found with them in foods. The reaction of the body is traumatic. Isolated from its natural context in a food, sodium chloride acts like a drug rather than a food. Practitioners of the drugless healing arts commonly use the organic, biochemical sodium contained in natural foods to reverse the conditions brought on by excessive intake of inorganic sodium.

Sodium is needed by many tissues, particularly the synovial membranes of the joints, cartilage, ligaments, the liver, the spleen, muscles, the stomach wall, the brain, blood corpuscles, and interstitial fluid. When persons lack adequate supplies of sodium from organic sources and receive too much sodium from inorganic sources, they become prone to developing arthritic conditions—inflammation of the joints. Excess sodium changes the chemistry of the joint fluids, irritating the membranes and allowing calcium to precipitate from a solution, causing deposits and spurs. These conditions frequently can be treated successfully with an increased intake of foods that are naturally high in organic sodium. Because sodium is such an important and copious electrolyte in the body, and because much of it can be easily lost via perspiration caused by heavy physical work, active participation in sports, sitting in a sauna, and so on, people require organic-sodium replacement.

One of my patients was a prominent basketball player. He had four operations to repair torn cartilage in his ankle. When this big, six-foot one-inch man came to me, I said, "You know, you haven't fed that ankle."

"What do you mean I haven't fed that ankle?" he asked.

"That joint material needs sodium, the type of sodium contained in foods, in order to repair and rejuvenate."

When I asked him how much weight he loses when playing a game, he replied, "As much as fifteen pounds." What do you suppose constitutes those fifteen pounds he loses? Water and salt. Half of salt is sodium. Sodium is the predominant mineral lost through perspiration. He needed extra organic sodium to replace the lost sodium and to help repair his injured tissues. Hot, humid weather, excessive water consumption, and perspiration deplete sodium salts rapidly. Heavy physical work and active sports demand a liberal organic-sodium diet, as do fevers, saunas, extreme excitement, and passion.

Replacement sodium should come from the organic salts of fruits and vegetables, not from salt tablets or other inorganic sources. Foods naturally rich in sodium possess an organic, biochemical, easily assimilated form of sodium, whereas common table salt, many food additives and preservatives, and other chemicalized "foods" manufactured in the laboratory and sold in stores contain inorganic sodium that is not compatible with the human body.

It is important to know the difference between chemical, inorganic table salt and the biochemical, organic sodium found in natural foods. Too many people disregard the distinction between inorganic salt and the biochemical sodium in organic foods. Organic sodium neutralizes acetic, butyric, lactic, and fatty acids, which are the byproducts of an excessive intake of fatty, starchy foods, meat, lard, butter, potatoes, oily nuts, and many other foods. In so doing, sodium from organic foods works gently and consistently, without undesirable side effects.

There are many salt substitutes on the market that are a mixture of garden herbs. These are naturally occurring vegetable salts that have a salty taste. Vegetable salts may be used as seasonings along with natural spices to enhance the flavors of foods. These vegetable salts are biochemical salts and cause no harm to the body.

The Excessive Consumption of Sugar

Sixty years ago, the average person in the United States consumed an estimated 16 pounds of refined sugar a year. That figure has been steadily rising until today it stands at 125 pounds. That's an increase of approximately 800 percent!

Organic foods such as vegetables, fruits, honey, and grains are easily metabolized by the body. Refined foods such as white sugar do not meet the body's nutritional needs and provide no more than a pleasing taste with empty calories. Aside from producing a quick burst of energy, refined sugar has only harmful effects on the body.

Among other things, it promotes tooth decay and leaches calcium from the body, destroying the delicate balance between calcium and phosphorus.

Excess white sugar also contributes to hypoglycemia (low blood sugar), a condition caused primarily by a diet high in refined carbohydrates. Eating refined sugar causes insulin to be released from the pancreas, which signals the liver to convert blood sugar to glycogen for storage. The body quickly uses up the glucose from the refined sugar, and the liver simply cannot break down the glycogen again fast enough to restore a normal blood-sugar level. Low blood sugar can contribute to or trigger nervousness, fatigue, headaches, asthma, alcoholism, and epileptic seizures. Indirectly, the consumption of white sugar contributes to all the diseases caused by a deficiency of protein, minerals, or vitamins. Many people fill up on sugar and then do not eat foods that supply the necessary nutrients.

It is interesting to note that alcohol and refined sugar have much in common. Both alcohol and refined sugar can be addictive. Both cause similar metabolic processes in the body. Both deplete the body of its stores of vitamins and minerals. Both cause mood swings and uncontrolled personality changes. Both contribute to degenerative diseases. Addiction to both decreases interest in nourishing foods, the very thing that helps to control the addictions.

Healthy substitutes for refined sugar include the more crudely refined date and fruit sugars, molasses, pure maple syrup, and raw, unheated honey. However, people with a sweet tooth should be careful not to consume any sugars in excess. Be aware that many of the foods you consume give you a hefty dose of sugar.

The Excessive Consumption of Wheat

Television and the rest of the mass media have for many years treated wheat as the most-favored breakfast. Wheat is also a prime ingredient in breads, waffles, pies, and pastries. It has earned a regular place at the dining table morning, noon, and night, and is a time-honored snack given to children in the form of cakes, crackers, and cookies. In the American diet, 29 percent of food intake each day is wheat. This is an outrageous amount of wheat consumption! Wheat should compose about 6 percent of the diet, not 29 percent.

When used in excess, the staff of life can cause many serious health problems. Wheat contains gluten, the sticky substance responsible for the elasticity in bread dough. Unfortunately, gluten also adheres to the bowel in the same sticky manner. Some people are very sensitive to gluten, so much so that they suffer a breakdown in their ileum. When the ileum breaks down enough to cause problems with absorption, it is known as celiac disease.

Celiac disease is characterized by diarrhea, malnutrition, bleeding in the bowel, and hypocalcemia. Gluten-sensitive individuals must avoid foods containing gluten entirely in order to regain and maintain their health. Even people who are not genetically sensitive to gluten should avoid an excess of foods containing gluten. Spastic conditions and other bowel problems are related to gluten in the diet when it is consumed in excess. Excessive wheat intake is also considered to be a factor in the formation of diverticula. In any case, greens and other vegetables assist in restoring the ileum to normal function.

The modern refining techniques of milling, polishing, processing, and bleaching destroy wheat's important biochemical elements. At the same time, the starch remains intact. Vitamin E, which helps to normalize heart function, is found in the wheat germ, a part of the kernel's outside covering that is removed in the refining process.

Instead of focusing on wheat, try other grains. Excellent substitutes include rye, millet, corn, and rice, which do not contain gluten and are high in nutritional value. All are available as whole grains and flour, as well as bread, cereal, and other products.

THE NINE DIETARY LAWS

In addition to avoiding the six nutritional sins, you should follow the nine dietary laws. The same as the nutritional sins, the dietary laws concern the foods you eat. Eating the proper foods in the proper amounts and prepared using proper methods will help you regain and maintain a state of optimum health. The nine dietary laws include the Law of Natural, Pure, and Whole; the Law of Proportions; the Law of Acid-Alkaline Balance; the Law of Variety; the Law of Raw Foods; the Law of Natural Cure; the Law of Moderation; the Law of Deficiency; and the Law of Food Combining. (For a quick description of these laws, see "The Dietary Laws at a Glance" on page 169.)

Dietary Law Number One: The Law of Natural, Pure, and Whole

The word "health" comes from an old Teutonic word meaning "salvation." If good health is part of salvation, the foods we eat have to be natural, pure, and whole.

What God makes for us is natural. You cannot pickle a cucumber and make it better than God made it originally. You can't bleach

The Dietary Laws at a Glance

Following are the nine dietary laws that all people should heed to reach and maintain optimum health:

❑ *Dietary Law Number One: The Law of Natural, Pure, and Whole.* Our foods should be natural, whole, and pure. Whole foods build a whole body.

❑ *Dietary Law Number Two: The Law of Proportions.* We should eat foods in the proper proportions. Each day we should have six vegetables, two fruits, one starch, and one protein.

❑ *Dietary Law Number Three: The Law of Acid-Alkaline Balance.* Our diets should be 80-percent alkaline and 20-percent acid. Vegetables and fruits are alkaline. Starches and proteins are acid.

❑ *Dietary Law Number Four: The Law of Variety.* Our diets should have the proper variety. Each day we should eat different vegetables, different fruits, different starches, and different proteins.

❑ *Dietary Law Number Five: The Law of Raw Foods.* Our diets should be 60-percent raw foods. The natural, raw form of foods provides the most nutritional value. They supply the best vitamins, minerals, and live enzymes.

❑ *Dietary Law Number Six: The Law of Natural Cure.* Nature cures, but she must be given the opportunity. Only when we eat properly is the body supplied with the nutrients nature needs to accomplish tissue repair and replacement.

❑ *Dietary Law Number Seven: The Law of Moderation.* We cannot eat one or a few foods to excess without causing nutritional deficiencies due to the lack of variety in the diet.

❑ *Dietary Law Number Eight: The Law of Deficiency.* If we do not eat enough of the right foods, we will develop nutritional deficiencies. Every disease is associated with some kind of nutritional deficiency.

❑ *Dietary Law Number Nine: The Law of Food Combining.* Certain starches and proteins—for example, meat and potatoes, and eggs and hash browns—should not be eaten together. It is all right to put milk on cooked oatmeal or millet. Eat melons separately from other foods.

For a complete discussion of these dietary laws, see "The Nine Dietary Laws" on page 168.

whole-wheat flour and make it better than God made. If God made it for human beings to eat, I don't think anyone can improve on it.

Whenever humans alter a food, they nearly always do something that reduces its value. Through processing, salting, bleaching, heating, and preserving, we create foods so altered that we have every reason to fear their effects on the our bodies.

One example of an unnatural food is cyclamate. Introduced some years ago as a sugar substitute, cyclamate was found to cause cancer in laboratory animals and thus was banned by the FDA. Saccharin, another sugar substitute, was also found to be linked to cancer, but Congress overruled an FDA attempt to ban it because of objections from diabetics and manufacturers. Now there is aspartame, another chemical sweetener, and time will tell what its side effects are. Already there is evidence that some people experience headache pain after using aspartame. Even white sugar is not a natural food because it has been through a refining process that removed all its vitamins and minerals. Some common natural sweeteners are honey, bee pollen, maple syrup, unrefined sugar-cane juice, natural rice syrup, molasses, and fruit.

My nutritional program is based on foods that are pure. Sprayed foods are not pure. A food cannot be called pure unless it was organically grown in a soil that was not chemicalized with artificial fertilizer. Foods also cannot be called pure if they were pickled, salted, processed, or canned. Many canned and packaged foods have labels that show the chemicals that were added. None of these are pure foods. Stay away from these foods as much as you possibly can. Avoid additives during cooking. Some restaurants add monosodium glutamate (MSG) to their food. Some people have allergic reactions to MSG.

Fruits and vegetables are among the purest foods we can get, yet we have to be careful to wash them thoroughly. Not only do they possibly have pesticide-spray residues on them, but they are often sprayed with sulfite chemicals to help them stay fresh looking, green, and crisp, especially on salad bars. Many people are allergic to sulfite sprays, and a number of people have died after eating sulfite-sprayed food.

We cannot live on altered or depleted food. Eating such food will eventually cause deficiency problems. I first learned about this when I studied the work of Professor E.V. McCollum of Johns Hopkins University. Dr. McCollum removed the calcium from the food he gave to his research animals and found that the animals could not develop good bones. He discovered that if he removed the potassium from the food, the animals didn't develop good muscles. Many of the processed foods people eat lack essential nutrients, nutrients that may have been present in the food prior to its processing, but were destroyed, either by mechanical means or by the high heat associated with many processing methods. Milk is a good example. As mentioned earlier in this chapter, raw milk contains enzymes such as phosphatase, which is essential for calcium absorption. Without phosphatase, which is destroyed by the heat of pasteurization, much of the calcium in pasteurized milk cannot be absorbed.

The destruction of phosphatase in pasteurized milk and products made from it is believed to be the chief reason for the increase in osteoporosis and in the resulting fractured hips among the elderly. Pasteurized dairy products are, nonetheless, heavily advertised for their high calcium content. People who consume nutritionally depleted foods over an extended period of time develop deficiency problems unless they make up for the deficiency in some way.

Deficiency problems were uncovered in a Dutch study in Java in the 1890s. Chickens fed only white rice for a couple of months developed a condition called droop wing. They couldn't hold their wings up. If they had continued eating only the white rice, the chickens would have died. However, the chickens with droop wing were instead fed whole-grain brown rice, and they recovered. In a similar experiment, pigeons fed white rice lost strength in their legs and became unable to stand. Given rice polishings to eat, they recovered enough strength in a matter of a few hours to walk around. Even near the point of death, pigeons were revived by being fed rice polishings. The disease that causes droop wing in chickens and loss of leg strength in pigeons was found to be beriberi, a vitamin-B_1 deficiency, the first deficiency disease discovered.

White sugar, white flour, and white rice are all examples of refined foods, foods depleted of some or all vitamins, minerals, and fiber. I call these foods "excoriated, foodless substances," because they no longer deserve to be called "foods." Eating such foods results in deficiencies in the body, and deficiencies create conditions that lead to disease.

It has been reported that the refining of whole-wheat flour reduces some twenty-seven elements to a minimum. In other words, we are cheated out of many nutrients that our bodies need. The thyroid breaks down from lack of iodine, the bones and teeth from lack of calcium, the muscle tissue from lack of potassium. By having whole food, we build a whole body. Can you understand now why some parts of your body may be underfed and other parts overfed? That's what happens in many different diseases in which certain organs break down from a lack of required chemical elements.

When I discuss whole foods, I include whole cereal grains, fruits, vegetables, whole milk, nuts, and seeds. However, I include milk with some caution because it is usually pasteurized. We should be able to get raw milk from cows that are milked under sanitary conditions, with the whole process subject to ongoing health and cleanliness inspections. We should be willing to pay a few extra cents a quart to get certified raw whole milk because it is much better for us. We cannot live on depleted and altered food alone.

I once received a letter from a man who had Perthes' disease. In Perthes' disease, holes develop in the hip portion of the femur, the large bone of the thigh. Perthes' disease is usually seen in young males between the ages of four and ten. This man, though, was fifty-six years of age, and his doctor had told him that it's very difficult—almost impossible—to cure Perthes' disease at this age. But the man said that after following my food regimen for a year and a half, his femur became much better. Is this possible? Yes, I often see food replenishing the chemical needs of the body. Good health begins with my first dietary law—food should be natural, pure, and whole.

Most of our foods today are what I call "dollar foods." The majority of people who produce foods for us know practically nothing about health. They are in business only for profit, and yet they are feeding us. I have only to look at the average family to know that things must change. Today's parents are raising doctors' bills. Their children are future doctors' bills. There's no reason for all this ill-health among our children. We can reduce our doctors' bills by learning what are the right foods to give our children.

The average doctor is not going to teach you about bowel care, nutrition, exercise, or right living. He has a treatment that he's trained to give. He's going to give you something—a shot or a prescription—to take care of your symptoms regardless of your bad habits, poor nutrition, or enervating lifestyle. He and the pharmacist are going to make their living on your ignorance. But we can't just point our fingers at doctors. Many patients are also to blame because they want the doctor to give them something that will allow them to go on living the same way they have been living. They don't realize that their bad habits caused their sickness in the first place. We would do well to remember that whenever we point a finger at someone, we have three fingers pointing back at us!

Doctors make a living on your living—that is, on the way you live your life. They make a living on your ignorance, and I think it's time for people to wake up and recognize that if they make the move to natural, pure, and whole foods, they will make the biggest and best change that can be made.

Dietary Law Number Two: The Law of Proportions

The second dietary law is that we have to eat the various types of foods—vegetables, fruits, starches, and proteins—in the proper proportions. This proper-proportion law is lovely! After all, the human body is composed of just the right proportions of calcium, silicon, iodine, and the other minerals. We couldn't survive by consuming all the minerals in equal amounts. We need to feed our bodies the correct proportions.

Every day we should have six vegetables, two fruits, one good-quality starch, and one good-quality protein. There are people who get carried away with dietary extremes, but I favor a more middle-of-the-road approach. Because I believe that getting well and staying healthy should be a cooperative effort between patient and doctor, I don't want to work with you if you choose to go to the extreme of not eating any protein. I do not want to work with you if you don't want to allow yourself a good starch. These are extremes. I don't want to work with you if you insist on eliminating all fruits or vegetables from your diet. And, I can't work with you if you don't agree to consume your foods in the correct proportions. Heaven knows, I believe in good eliminations! But you can't go to the extreme of eliminating so many foods from your diet that you throw the necessary proportions way off balance and still expect to be well. You see, I don't like to have failures in my work. I am a person who thrives on success. I feel successful when I see my patients get well. And you cannot successfully get well if you neglect the Law of Proportions.

In the dietary plan I recommend, called the Health and Harmony Food Regimen, there is a harmonious balance among the foods that takes care of about 95 percent of people. (For a complete description of the Health and Harmony Food Regimen, see page 192.) Almost all the people who come to me can follow my dietary plan and meet their nutritional needs. I realize that most things in life are not suitable for every person, so I say "95 percent," not "100 percent."

With the right foods in the right proportions, your body will make improvements day by day, slowly, definitely, so that at the end of six months, you will have a better body without going from one diet to another. However, you don't have to worry about perfection in this proportion business. If you divide your recommended starch intake between two meals instead of consuming it all at one meal, you will be all right. If you divide your recommended protein intake between two meals instead of having it all in one, I think you'll be fine. On the other hand, you shouldn't consume one and one-half pounds of steak just because you're having all your protein at one meal. I'm exaggerating to make a point. People often have problems when they consume too much starch or protein. However, people do not seem to have any problems when they eat large quantities of vegetables and fruits.

Dietary Law Number Three: The Law of Acid-Alkaline Balance

It is very important for you to understand that the foods you eat should be 80-percent alkaline and 20-percent acid. It is important to eat more alkaline foods because the acid wastes produced in the body need to be neutralized. The acid-alkaline balance of the blood (blood pH) is controlled largely by the respiratory system and the kidneys, with complex chemical buffering actions preventing sudden deviations. However, it is food that provides the continuous supply of the major minerals—calcium, potassium, sodium, and magnesium—that compose the foundation of the acid-neutralizing bases. The acid-producing foods are proteins, starches, and sugars.

On my Health and Harmony Food Regimen, you will eat six vegetables, two fruits, one starch, and one protein each day. (I left out sugars because you're not supposed to eat them!) Vegetables and fruits should amount to eight of every ten of the foods you eat. This makes the diet 80-percent alkaline. Starches and proteins should add up to two of every ten of the foods you eat, making the diet

20-percent acid. You are responsible for taking portions of the right sizes to make the percentages come out approximately right.

Here is the problem: United States government figures show that the average American diet contains only 20-percent fruits and vegetables, and the National Academy of Sciences tells us that the average diet has about twice as much fat as it should. It is, therefore, my conservative estimate that the average diet is probably at least 50- to 60-percent acid-forming foods. That is something to think about, especially in view of today's major health problems.

Dietary Law Number Four: The Law of Variety

We need to eat the proper variety of foods. But what is the proper variety? My aunt always had vegetables, but only carrots and peas. She never had any other vegetables. Some people insist on eating prunes at every breakfast. Every morning, they're full of prunes. Avocados are wonderful, but not morning, noon, and night, week in and week out. You can't have just potatoes every day either. People who eat like this restrict their foods so much that they produce a one-sided body. Your body can work only with what you give it. Variety ensures that your body gets all the elements it needs.

Variety is important for many reasons. The same food item is different in different parts of the country. For example, apples from the state of Washington are significantly different from California apples. Celery from Utah is different from New York celery. This is because these foods are grown in different soils. Different soils have different mineral contents, and that affects the mineral content of the produce. As a result, celery grown in New York has 25-percent less sodium than celery grown in the Salt Lake Valley of Utah. When plants are grown in a salty soil, they have a higher sodium content. Celery grown in the soil around Battle Creek, Michigan, has a higher sodium content than celery grown in most other areas of the country. So, in addition to different kinds of food, the Law of Variety also applies to the type of soil in which food is grown.

The average American diet is 54-percent wheat and milk products, and 9-percent sugar. This violates the Law of Variety. We need fruits, vegetables, whole grains, nuts, seeds, and legumes in our diets, and we need variety in our proteins, starches, and fats—that is, a much greater variety than we are now getting. When you seek variety in your diet, you need to do so on a day-by-day and week-by-week basis. What you have today, you shouldn't have tomorrow. You should have different foods from day to day. Why should your salad dressing always be oil, honey, and lemon? Why can't you have a buttermilk dressing? Why can't you have a cheese dressing or an avocado dressing? You don't need to have the same thing every day or even four days a week. When you do, you are eating out of habit, and a good deal of our diet problems come from habits in our eating. The English drink tea all the time, and they suffer more from rheumatism than any other culture in the world. Because the English add a good deal of sugar to their tea, they aggravate their rheumatic conditions. Sugar robs the body of sodium, which neutralizes the acids associated with the condition. I call these acids "rheumatic acids" because they irritate the joints.

Once I visited Heliconia, a little town in South America where the people died at the average age of twenty-nine. The diet there was limited to sugar cane and corn. In an experiment conducted by the Upjohn Company, a major American pharmaceutical firm, soy powder was added to the diet. The average life span rapidly increased to thirty-nine. This ten-year increase occurred just because a little protein was added to the diet. This story certainly illustrates what can happen if a diet seriously lacks variety.

Dietary Law Number Five: The Law of Raw Foods

I believe that 60 percent of the food we eat each day should be raw. I used to say 50 percent, but I found that people cheat a little. They don't eat all the raw foods they should, so I raised my recommendation to 60 percent. In addition to vitamins and minerals, raw foods supply the natural enzymes needed by the human body. The high temperatures associated with cooking and processing destroy these enzymes. When you eat 60 percent of your foods raw, you also tend to get the proper balance of water.

Raw foods also supply the fiber that is so necessary for good health. Raw vegetables are the best sources of fiber. You cannot live on soup, soft foods, creamy sauces, and the like, and expect your intestinal tract to work properly. Earlier in this chapter, I discussed the importance of fiber in the daily diet. But did you know that one of the best ways to obtain the fiber you need is to eat raw fruits and vegetables, whole grains, nuts, and seeds? If you eat these foods, you won't have to chase the "bran wagon," one of the latest fiber fads.

As I have already mentioned, government figures show that the average American diet includes about 20-percent fruits and vegetables. Raw nuts and seeds are not included in the figures because they probably amount to less than 0.1 percent. Many people eat none at all.

We should eat more raw nuts and seeds, as well as seed and nut butters, and we should drink seed- and nut-milk beverages instead of dairy products. We should drink raw vegetable and fruit juices, or health cocktails made from a variety of blended ingredients, at least twice a day. Most families consume more cooked vegetables than raw vegetables, but we need to have at least two large salads a day, with each salad containing five to eight raw ingredients.

Although it is sometimes necessary to go to extremes to accomplish a specific purpose, it is usually not safe or desirable to linger there. Extremism should not be a way of life. Some people go to extremes with raw foods. They "go to the edges," as they say in London. Some people eat only raw foods, while others are fruitarians, living entirely on fruit. Although raw foods are good, I am not suggesting that you follow an extreme raw diet, eating nearly all your foods raw. I would rather you follow a middle path. Even eating 60 percent of your foods raw, as I prefer, may take a period of time to get used to. My advice is to take it slowly, building up to 60 percent over a few months' time.

When I treat people who have been on refined foods and overcooked foods for twenty years, I have to make up for the deficiencies that resulted. I want to correct the problems as quickly as possible, and the Health and Harmony Food Regimen accomplishes this well. In most cases, it takes at least a year to see changes in the body. You think that's slow? On the contrary, that's pretty fast! You can't destroy your body just by consuming the wrong foods for a week. Likewise, you can't expect to build your body up again by eating well for just a week. I once had a woman say to me, "I had a salad last week, and I didn't notice any difference." I wonder about her expectations. But if you follow through, you'll see some lovely things happen.

Dietary Law Number Six: The Law of Natural Cure

Nature cures, but we must give her the opportunity. Nature cures if we get out of her way. There may be things we can do to assist her, but most of the time, we just have to learn how to stop thwarting her healing process. If you don't get enough sleep, you can't be well. If your marriage is not good, you can't be well. If your job disturbs you, irritates you, you can't be well. But, whatever the particular circumstances of your life, *it is vital that you get the proper nutrition.* We can straighten out basically anything in life, but if we don't straighten out our nutrition, we cannot have good health. And with good health, we are better able to cope with the stresses of life.

Drug therapy, surgery, and radiation sometimes stop diseases, but more often than not, they simply drive the disease deeper into the tissues or cause it to move to some other organ or part of the body. Only by following nature's ways can we bring lasting healing and build good tissue. Only when the tissues are replaced is healing complete. The only true healing is natural healing, the only kind of healing that is able to bring full recovery to bodily tissues. You must learn how to cooperate with nature in order to be well.

Dietary Law Number Seven: The Law of Moderation

When we consume one or more foods in excess, we create an imbalance in the body. The imbalance caused by overeating in general results in obesity. One person who violated the Law of Moderation was Orson Welles, the famous Hollywood film genius, whose weight reached four hundred pounds from overeating before he died on October 10, 1985. Welles was notorious for eating large beef-and-gravy dinners with lots of rolls and butter, finishing up with generous portions of dessert. Welles knew that his diabetes, heart condition, and circulatory problems made overeating especially dangerous, but he once told a friend, "The only thing that makes me happy is eating."

According to surveys, over 60 percent of Americans are overweight, with about 40 percent obese. This is due to excess, to overeating in general and to eating an imbalanced diet with an excess of only a few foods. An excess of any of the three major food categories—protein, carbohydrates, or fats—causes imbalance in the body and can contribute to obesity.

While it is almost impossible to overeat whole grains and fresh fruits and vegetables, most vegetarian diets warn against overeating because excessive consumption of any food will result in obesity and toxicity. Violating the Law of Moderation also creates a toxic body, as the systems of elimination are taxed. Excessive protein in the diet overtaxes the stomach, which may not have enough hydrochloric acid to break down the protein for complete digestion and assimilation in the small intestine. Undigested protein causes overgrowth of putrefactive bacteria in the bowel, which results in toxic byproducts such as indole, skatole, and acidic amines. These toxic substances enter the bloodstream, causing tissue damage and settling in inherently weak organs and tissues. Excess digested and assimilated protein is simply converted to fat and stored in the tissues.

Refined carbohydrates such as wheat products and white sugar make up 38 percent of the average American diet, an amount that is an unhealthy excess for two reasons. First, digestively, all it takes to break down refined carbohydrates into glucose for absorption is a single, rapid chemical step. If there is more simple sugar than the body needs, the excess sugar places a strain on the islands of Langerhans, the specialized pancreatic cells that produce insulin. Insulin is needed to transport glucose across cell membranes into cells, where it is oxidized to produce energy. It seems to me that excess sugar consumed over time can weaken the body's ability to produce insulin. When this happens, diabetes results. There are also genetic predispositions to diabetes that may be triggered by obesity, stress, pregnancy, menopause, or another factor. Uncontrolled diabetes produces an acidic condition called diabetic acidosis, which may lead to coma. Second, excess sugar is stored in liver and muscle tissue as glycogn for use when reserves are needed. When all the glycogen storage sites are full, the remaining sugar is converted to fat.

Because they form acid products as they are metabolized, white sugar, white-flour products, and all other processed carbohydrates alter the pH balance of the body. They rob the body of its reserve of alkalinizing elements—mainly calcium, sodium, and potassium—which neutralize the unnatural acidic substances. If the body is robbed of calcium, sodium, and potassium, the bones, teeth, joints, and all the other tissues in the body are adversely affected. Some researchers have pointed out that white bread and many other white-flour baked goods also contribute to a sluggish bowel and constipation, allowing the assimilation of toxic material through the bowel wall.

As I already mentioned, the average American diet contains twice as much fat as the National Academy of Sciences recommends. Excess fat stresses the liver and gallbladder, promotes obesity, and contributes to diabetes, cardiovascular disease (arteriosclerosis and atherosclerosis), and cancer. An excess of any food taxes the kidneys as they strive to remove the resultant acids and toxic waste products from the blood. Furthermore, if we eat an excess of some foods, we may not eat the other foods we need, which can lead to nutritional deficiencies. Another consequence of excess is tissue irritation and catarrh. Allergies, colds, and catarrhal troubles are more common in persons who eat too much of a certain food. We find that 63 percent of the average American diet is made up of milk, wheat, and sugar. This is far too much. It should be closer to 12 percent.

Another excess in the average diet is meat and potatoes. Government studies have linked diets high in proteins and fats to cancer and heart disease. When we eat too much, especially proteins and starches, a greater amount of hydrochloric acid is needed in the stomach to prepare the food for digestion. If the amount of hydrochloric acid is insufficient, putrefaction, gas, and toxic conditions may develop in the bowel.

Eating in excess is self-abuse. So is undereating, which is starvation. We need to remember that disease preys on a malnourished body. We cannot upset the chemical balance of the body without eventually suffering serious consequences. We therefore need to know just how much to eat. If you eat a balanced diet and are overweight, you should take one-third (more or less) of each food on your plate and push it off to the side. When you cut back on food, don't just cut out starches. Don't just cut out proteins. Cut out part of your regular starch consumption, part of your regular protein consumption, part of your regular vegetable consumption, and part of your regular fruit comsumption. If you cut out a portion of everything, you retain the balance in your diet. To help reduce, eat a child's portion instead of a full plate. If you do a farmer's work, it is all right to have a farmer's big breakfast, because you'll work it off. However, this breakfast is not good for a person who sits at a desk all day. Such a person will gain weight, unless he or she has an unusually fast metabolism. Remember, insurance companies tell us that the smaller the waistline, the longer the lifeline.

Dietary Law Number Eight: The Law of Deficiency

The Law of Deficiency is a violation of the Law of Moderation, and this is hazardous. What you neglect to eat can affect your health just as much as what you do eat. You are violating the Law of Deficiency when:

❑ You are undernourished or starving.

❑ You use refined foods lacking vitamins and minerals.

❑ You use foods grown in depleted soils.

❑ You do not eat adequately for your job demands or daily stress levels.

❑ You consume an imbalanced or one-sided diet.

❑ You are deficient in one nutrient, vitamin, or mineral, or in many.

Remember, *every disease involves a nutritional deficiency*. Among the best-known diseases caused by nutritional deficiencies is beriberi, which is caused by vitamin-B_1 deficiency and is common among people who eat refined white rice. Osteoporosis, a bone-weakening disease, is epidemic among American women over the age of sixty and is due to mineral deficiencies. Kwashiorkor, common in Third World countries, is a disease resulting from protein deficiency. Not only are disease processes often preceded by nutritional deficiencies, but all diseases create deficiencies through their impact on the endocrine glands, metabolism, and blood chemistry.

Dietary Law Number Nine: The Law of Food Combining

Some people place a lot of importance on food combining. I do not. However, when you are ill and chronically fatigued, food combining becomes much more important. When you are sick or tired, your body doesn't have the energy to digest foods properly, and any additional digestive requirement becomes a liability. Even when you are well, you should make natural foods the priority. It's better to have natural foods in any combination than to have junk foods in perfect combinations.

Extreme starches and extreme proteins should not be consumed together. Examples are meat and potatoes, and eggs and hash browns, two common and very bad combinations. It is best not to have potatoes at all for breakfast, but I don't object to having protein and whole-grain cereals together. Nature doesn't do a perfect job of food combining. It's all right to eat a natural food that contains both starch and protein. However, just because nature formulates foods containing both protein and starch doesn't mean that we can consume an overwhelmingly protein food in large quantities at the same meal with a food that is predominately starch.

In addition, melons do not mix well with most other foods from a digestive standpoint and should be consumed separately. They make a wonderful between-meal snack. Ideally, sweet dried fruits should not be consumed with citrus fruits. While I fully recognize that some people have made a science of food combining, coming up with detailed charts and lists, I believe the combinations I just mentioned are the most important. It is my opinion that people who possess reasonably good digestive function need not concern themselves with food combining.

THE NECESSITY OF CHEMICAL BALANCE

If the laws of proper eating are followed, you will have chemical balance. One of the subtlest forms of bodily imbalance that I know of is the chemical, or nutritional, imbalance. Such an imbalance sneaks up so slowly that we don't see it coming. It can exist even before symptoms present themselves. Eventually, a chemical imbalance takes its toll. A chemical deficiency or imbalance is at the root of nearly every ill.

A healthy, well-functioning bowel contains sodium, potassium, and magnesium. These three chemical elements are sorely lacking in biochemical form in our modern foods. Sodium neutralizes acid and is required by the tissues that are pliable, active, and movable—that is, the joints, ligaments, and tendons. It is found in the lymphatic system, assists in the reconstruction of the bowel wall, and helps the bowel to regain pliability in its ligamentous support structures. Sodium neutralizes the gases of putrefaction and acts as a sweetener in the intestinal tract, much the same way that baking soda (sodium bicarbonate) "sweetens" the mouth when used to brush the teeth.

Potassium is necessary for the muscle structure and elasticity that speed transit time in the bowel. The same as sodium, it is needed to neutralize acids in the body. Potassium should always be supplied in the proper proportion to sodium. That proportion, according to Richard Passwater, Ph.D., is nine parts potassium to four parts sodium.

Magnesium, in association with calcium, relaxes the muscles of the body and helps hold potassium in the cells. It helps to eliminate spastic conditions, strictures, tension, disorders resulting from emotional strain, loss of tone, and ballooned conditions in the bowel. It acts like a laxative in the bowel and, therefore, is an essential element for good bowel movements. Milk of Magnesia, one of the more popular over-the-counter medications, is a good peristaltic stimulator. However, it contains an inorganic form of magnesium that gives only symptomatic relief, not natural and long-lasting correction. The same as inorganic substances in food, inorganic substances in medications do not act favorably in rebuilding bodily tissues. The biochemical, organic magnesium that occurs naturally in food is what does the greatest amount of good.

When these three important minerals—sodium, potassium, and magnesium—are lacking in the diet, they must be obtained from the tissues of the bowel wall, where they are stored. I believe that the bowel wall is one of the most maltreated structures of the body, functioning in a constant state of semistarvation for the biochemical elements it needs for day-to-day functioning. The most important elements found in the bowel wall must be kept in constant supply or the body suffers the consequences. The bowel can be rebuilt only if its primary chemical elements—sodium, potassium, and magnesium—are available.

Foods Rich in Sodium

The best organic source of sodium is whey, the watery part of milk that separates from the curds in the process of making cheese. Whey helps to return lactobacillus bacteria and other intestinal flora to the bowel.

Veal-joint broth and powdered whey made from cow's or goat's milk are concentrated sources of sodium. Goat's milk, whey, and black mission figs are a superior sodium combination (and also a champion arthritis remedy). Other high-sodium foods are:

❑ Apples

❑ Apricots, dried

❑ Asparagus

❑ Barley

❑ Beet greens

❑ Beets

❑ Black olives

❑ Carrots

❑ Celery

❑ Cheese

❑ Chickpeas, dried

❑ Coconut, dried

❑ Collard greens

❑ Dandelion greens

❑ Dates

❑ Dulse

❑ Egg yolks

❑ Figs

❑ Fish

❑ Goat's milk

❑ Horseradish

❑ Irish moss

❑ Kale

❑ Kelp

❑ Lentils

❑ Milk, raw

❑ Mustard greens

❑ Okra

❑ Parsley

❑ Peas, dried

❑ Prunes, dried

❑ Raisins

❑ Red cabbage

❑ Red peppers

❑ Sesame seeds

❑ Spinach

❑ Strawberries

❑ Sunflower seeds

❑ Swiss chard

❑ Turnips

Moderate sources of sodium include cabbages besides red cabbage, water chestnuts, garlic, dried peaches, radishes, broccoli, Brussels sprouts, and cashew nuts.

Foods Rich in Potassium

Sun-dried black olives and Potato Peeling Broth (see page 120) are two of the best sources of potassium. However, when making Potato Peeling Broth, be careful not to overheat the soup because potassium is destroyed by excessive heat. Potassium is usually absent from processed foods, since commercial food processing tends to use heats high enough to be destructive.

The best sources of potassium are organic foods. Following is a partial list of foods high in potassium:

❑ Almonds	❑ Jerusalem artichokes
❑ Anise seeds	❑ Kale
❑ Apple cider vinegar	❑ Kelp
❑ Apple peelings	❑ Leaf lettuce
❑ Apples	❑ Lentils
❑ Apricots, dried	❑ Lima beans, dried
❑ Bananas	❑ Olives
❑ Beans (red, pinto, white, mung, string), dried	❑ Parsley
	❑ Parsnips
❑ Beet greens	❑ Peaches, bitter
❑ Beets (red, yellow)	❑ Pears, dried
❑ Black cherries	❑ Pecans
❑ Blueberries	❑ Potato peelings
❑ Broccoli	❑ Raisins
❑ Brown cheese	❑ Rice bran
❑ Brussels sprouts	❑ Rice polishings
❑ Carrots	❑ Sesame seeds, whole
❑ Cashews	❑ Soybeans, dried
❑ Cucumbers	❑ Soymilk
❑ Currants	❑ Spinach
❑ Dates	❑ Sunflower seeds
❑ Dulse	❑ Swiss chard
❑ Egg white, beaten	❑ Tomatoes
❑ Escarole	❑ Turnips

❏ Figs, dried   ❏ Walnuts
❏ Fish   ❏ Watercress
❏ Goat's milk   ❏ Wheat bran
❏ Grapes   ❏ Wheat germ
❏ Green turtle

There are also a number of herbs that are good sources of potassium. They include catnip, hops, horsetail, nettle, plantain, red clover, sage, and skullcap.

Foods Rich in Magnesium

Magnesium is highest in certain nuts and whole grains. Unpolished rice has eleven times the magnesium content of polished rice, and rice polishings are an even more concentrated source of the mineral. Wheat germ is another high-magnesium food, and a good deal of magnesium can be found in salad vegetables. Salads were almost absent from our diets for many years, but—thankfully—made a comeback during the final decades of the twentieth century. Some additional foods that are high in magnesium are as follows:

❏ Apples   ❏ Lentils
❏ Apples, dried   ❏ Mint
❏ Apricots, dried   ❏ New Zealand spinach
❏ Avocados   ❏ Oats
❏ Bananas, dried   ❏ Okra
❏ Beans (white, lima,   ❏ Onion tops
  garbanzo, snap), dried   ❏ Parsley
❏ Beet greens   ❏ Peaches
❏ Beets   ❏ Peanuts
❏ Black walnuts   ❏ Pears, dried
❏ Brazil nuts   ❏ Pecans
❏ Brown rice   ❏ Pistachio nuts
❏ Cabbage   ❏ Prunes
❏ Cashews   ❏ Sorrel
❏ Coconuts   ❏ Soybeans, dried

❑ Comfrey leaves
❑ Dates
❑ Dulse
❑ Endive
❑ English walnuts
❑ Figs, dried
❑ Filberts
❑ Fish
❑ Gelatin
❑ Goat's milk
❑ Grapes
❑ Green pepper
❑ Hickory nuts
❑ Honey

❑ Soymilk
❑ Sunflower seeds
❑ Sweet yellow corn
❑ Swiss chard
❑ Tofu
❑ Turbot
❑ Turnip greens
❑ Veal-joint broth
❑ Watercress
❑ Whiting
❑ Whole rye
❑ Whole wheat
❑ Wild rice
❑ Yellow cornmeal

Magnesium is found most abundantly in yellow cornmeal. However, most commercial cornmeal has been milled and refined so much that it no longer contains the fiber from the corn kernel's outer covering, which at one time made yellow cornmeal one of the great laxatives and one of the greatest bowel-toning foods. But in spite of this shortcoming, I believe that everyone should have yellow cornmeal at least two mornings a week in order to get adequate amounts of magnesium.

IN CONCLUSION

You must readjust your taste buds and your thinking if you wish to live a healthy and productive life. You can avoid committing nutritional sins if you read labels before purchasing commercial foods and avoid all products that contain heated fats or oils. Begin preparing your own dishes, making sure that the ingredients you buy are as natural, pure, and whole as those you would grow yourself. Of course, it is sometimes difficult or even impossible to obtain the best, but you should make a reasonable effort to do so. Remember, too, the importance of fiber to bowel health, for bowel health influences the proper function of all the other organs in the body and, therefore, indirectly helps reduce cholesterol.

Chapter 8

Additional Techniques for Bowel Management

In the days when I had my sanitariums, bowel cleansing utilizing the colema system had not yet been developed. Of course, the bowel's role in health was recognized, but in those days, tissue cleansing was achieved using diet, exercise, and rest. Patients got well after adopting improved ways of living and eating.

Fasting is a time-honored method of cleansing the body and getting it on a track to improved health. At my sanitariums, people fasted in the effort to regain their health. I employed quite a few different fasts, from complete water fasts to partial fasts, as well as a variety of modified or limited diets for specific purposes, including mono-diets (single-food diets). My guests also learned about my Health and Harmony Food Regimen, which, unlike other diets, is not a regimen used temporarily for a specific purpose, but a general plan for continued use. Since I had a great deal of success with all these diets, I am presenting some of them here for those readers who cannot follow the Ultimate Tissue Cleansing Program. Please remember, however, that diet alone cannot produce results as rapidly as a total cleansing program can.

FASTS AND LIMITED DIETS

Wisdom is the ability to find alternatives. I believe that we need to use our mental faculties to come up with alternatives in life whenever they are called for. There are many elimination regimes, and they all have approximately the same results because the body is given less food, simpler foods in simpler combinations, and foods containing more water to aid elimination. Any of the following regimes, if faithfully followed, will bring you excellent results. These fasts and limited diets are the Eleven-Day Elimination Diet, the One-Day-a-Week Fast, the Grape Fast, the Watermelon Flush, the Carrot-Juice Fast, and the Master Chlorophyll Elimination Diet.

The Eleven-Day Elimination Diet

Most people in good general health who want to overcome an average physical disorder can follow the Eleven-Day Elimination Diet. Persons who are weak or feeble, however, should not follow the plan for the full eleven days without supervision. Individuals with tuberculosis, bleeding from the bowel, or colitis should have both supervision and assistance. The length of time and the manner in which the foods are taken can be adjusted to suit the history of the patient. For instance, fruits, vegetables, and broths may be eaten for one day; fruit alone may be eaten for one day; or vegetables alone may be eaten for one to three days.

During the Eleven-Day Elimination Diet, you should take a hot bath every night. Take enemas, not colemas, during the first four or five days, then discontinue them to allow for natural movements. For the first three days, ingest nothing but water and fruit juices, preferably grapefruit juice. Drink one glass of juice every four hours. For the next two days, eat only fruit—grapes, melons, tomatoes, pears, peaches, plums, dried fruit (prunes, figs, and peaches) that has been rehydrated (see Appendix A), and baked apples. During the final six days, have tree-ripened citrus fruits for breakfast; a salad of three to six vegetables and two cups of Vital Broth for lunch; and two or three steamed vegetables and two cups of Vital Broth for dinner. (For a recipe for Vital Broth, see page 139.) If you become hungry between meals, you can have any kind of fruit or fruit juice. You can also drink fruit juice before retiring, if you wish. At every meal, eat plenty, but not to satiety. Rigid adherence to the diet is an absolute necessity if you desire to regain good health.

The One-Day-a-Week Fast

There are a host of ways in which to fast. Many people like to fast one day a week. When fasting this way, you can follow a juice diet or a fruit diet on that day. It is important to consume fresh, clean water during any fast. Water helps flush the toxins out of the body. A good regimen is to drink one-half glass of water every one and a half hours throughout the day. You will need more water on hot days, since you will perspire more. Be sure not to take big gulps of water, which should be cool, but never ice cold.

Although fasting is the quickest way using diet to encourage elimination in the body and the fastest way to move toxic materials out, rest is complementary to it. I believe that rest is one of the essentials for cure because it allows the body to regain the vitality it needs to throw off toxic materials and to eliminate the debris that has accumulated over a period of years. When you fast, you will need complete rest, physical and psychological. As you let your body rest, you will develop more tone and vitality than you could using any other procedure.

On the day that you fast, you should take an enema, not a colema, to empty the lower bowel. If you want to exercise a little, I recommend walking. Walk on level ground, and do not walk to the point of tiring. If you live in a cold climate, walk in a shopping mall or other warm place to avoid becoming chilled. It is important when fasting not to do anything to the point of fatigue.

The Grape Fast

On the Grape Fast, you should eat four pounds of grapes a day, averaging one pound every three hours. The grapes should have seeds, since fruits with seeds are more vital than fruits without seeds. People today eat too many hybrid foods including seedless grapes. The foods that nature originally gave us are the most vital foods. Concord, Fresno Beauty, Muscat, and red grapes are all good grapes for this diet.

In addition to grapes with seeds being preferable for this diet because they are more vital than grapes without seeds, the tartaric acid that surrounds grape seeds helps to eliminate catarrh. You do not need to swallow the seeds, but you should chew them finely to make sure you get all the tartar off the seeds. When chewing the grape skins, you'll find they are very bitter. The bitter taste is caused by the high level of potassium they contain. Potassium is a great alkalizer and cleanser in the body.

Especially at the beginning of the Grape Fast, you should take enemas, not colemas. Toxic materials will accumulate, and you'll need to keep everything moving along.

You can go on the Grape Fast for five to ten days without any supervision, but if you stay on the diet any longer, you should seek the guidance of someone who is competent in managing the diet. That person should be able to help you if you have a reaction that is strange to you. Many times, such a reaction is nothing more than a healing crisis or an elimination process.

The Watermelon Flush

The watermelon season presents an excellent opportunity for a good elimination diet. Watermelon is a wonderful diuretic, and eating watermelon exclusively helps to rid the colon of a lot of debris. In addition, the extra water picks up toxic materials and carries them off via the kidneys.

To follow the Watermelon Flush, simply eat watermelon in place of your regular fare at every meal. Follow this eating plan for three, four, or five days.

The Carrot-Juice Fast

I don't think there is any particular juice that will cure any specific disease, but many of my patients have benefited greatly from carrot juice. I believe that the rest a simple mono-diet affords the body, especially the digestive system, gives the body the opportunity to reverse any diseases that may be present and recover its health. It's the rest from food that does the trick. The elimination of food mixtures and the reduced demands made on the digestive and elimination systems help to overcome disease.

The Carrot-Juice Fast involves drinking eight ounces of carrot juice every three hours, more often if you like. You can do this for ten days, twenty days, or even longer. (Longer fasts, however, should always be supervised by a doctor.) One of my patients was on the Carrot-Juice Fast for a whole year. This is a long time to have nothing but carrot juice! It is an extreme. Although I don't like to go to extremes, sometimes it is necessary to accomplish a purpose. This man had an extreme condition of the bowel, but through the Carrot-Juice Fast, he got rid of it. The man passed mucous from his bowel with great frequency. His nearly continual eliminations were almost unbelievable. Sometimes they were even black. They consisted simply of accumulated, chronic, toxic material that he had to get rid of.

The Master Chlorophyll Elimination Diet

Liquid chlorophyll is an excellent addition to the daily diet. Furthermore, taking liquid chlorophyll every three hours for three or four days is a wonderful prelude to fasting. I consider chlorophyll to be the master cleanser for catarrhal conditions. Catarrh is best eliminated from the body through the use of greens. Liquid chlorophyll usually is extracted from alfalfa leaves and is high in potassium and iron.

The Master Chlorophyll Elimination Diet consists of just plain water and chlorophyll. Every three hours for three to four days, drink eight ounces of water, preferably distilled, to which one teaspoon of liquid chlorophyll has been added. If you wish, you can substitute vegetable juice for the water. Do not consume any other foods or beverages.

BREAKING A FAST OR LIMITED DIET

When breaking a fast or limited diet, do not immediately plunge into a regular diet. The longer you have been on the fast or limited diet, the more time you should allow yourself to ease back to eating full meals on a regular schedule. Plan on an average of two to six days. In addition, one or two days before concluding your fast or limited diet, discontinue taking enemas. This is to work toward natural bowel movements.

To break a fast on which you took nothing by mouth except water for about a week, do not consume anything but either vegetable or fruit juice for the first one or two days following the conclusion of the fast. Drink one eight-ounce glass of juice every three hours.

For breakfast and lunch on the third day following the fast, have oranges that have been peeled and sliced. The meat of an orange is one of the finest foods for the bowel. If you do not want to eat oranges, you can substitute finely shredded carrot that has been wilted by steaming for one minute. Both oranges and carrots help clean out toxic materials. For dinner on the third day, you may have a small green salad.

On the fourth day following the fast, add an eight-ounce glass of juice at 10 A.M. and another at 3 P.M. On the fifth day, you can have any fresh fruit for breakfast, along with an eight-ounce glass of vegetable or noncitrus-fruit juice. Have another eight-ounce glass of juice at 10 A.M. For lunch, you can have a small salad and a glass of juice, and at 3 P.M., you can have another glass of juice. For dinner, you can have a salad, one cooked vegetable, and juice. On the sixth day, you can add an egg or a tablespoon of nut butter to breakfast, and an extra vegetable to lunch and to dinner. On the seventh day, you will be ready to resume a regular diet. For a simple guideline to help you determine what to include in your regular diet, see "Bulk, Lubrication, and Moisture" on page 192.

I recommend following the Health and Harmony Food Regimen as your regular diet. If you followed a fast or limited diet, however, I recommend easing into it even if you break the fast as just described. On the first day, follow the Health and Harmony Food Regimen as outlined, but omit the starches and proteins. On the second day, add the starches. On the third day, add the proteins.

THE HEALTH AND HARMONY FOOD REGIMEN

Unlike most diets, the Health and Harmony Food Regimen is neither temporary nor remedial. Following it should become a habit. When the Health and Harmony Food Regimen is part of your everyday life, you won't need to think much about your vitamin, mineral, or caloric intake. Most diets are intended for a specific purpose, such as weight loss, cleansing, or avoiding allergic reactions. Often, these diets are a bit extreme and usually temporary. After accomplishing the purpose, the dieter usually returns to his or her regular way of eating. In contrast, the Health and Harmony Food Regimen is for continuous use. It is inclusive enough to fulfill all of the body's usual and customary needs. It is not a fad diet. Fad diets may not be harmful for temporary use, but many are limited and lopsided, and do not meet the body's needs over an extended period.

The Health and Harmony Food Regimen actually begins before

Bulk, Lubrication, and Moisture

Here is a simple guideline to keep in mind when considering whether to consume a certain food: Your food should in some way contribute to the bulk, lubrication, and moisture (BLM) in your bowel. Bulk, lubrication, and moisture combine to create an ideal bowel environment. Bulk creates the mass whereby good evacuation is assured. Lubrication allows an easy flow of materials through the digestive tract all the way to the anus. And moisture prevents the drying out of feces and the development of constipation.

If a food item does not contribute to BLM, don't eat it!

breakfast. Upon arising, at least one-half hour before your first meal of the day, drink four to six ounces of any natural, unsweetened fruit juice such as grape, pineapple, prune, fig, apple, or black-cherry juice. If desired, you can substitute a glass of warm water containing one teaspoon of liquid chlorophyll. Another option is a drink made of broth and lecithin. To make this drink, simply dissolve one teaspoon of vegetable-broth powder and one tablespoon of lecithin granules in a glass of warm water and stir.

After drinking your morning juice, but before eating breakfast, skin brush. (See "Skin Brushing" on page 118.) When you finish skin brushing, you should spend some time exercising, deep breathing, or playing. Then shower, starting with warm water and gradually lowering it until your breath quickens from the coolness. Never shower immediately upon arising. Finally, have your breakfast.

Breakfast

For breakfast every day, you should have a little fruit, one starch, and a healthy beverage. When possible, eat fruit in season. Good choices are melon, grapes, peaches, pears, berries, and apples. If you wish, you can sprinkle the fruit with some ground nuts or garnish it with a pat of nut butter. If fresh fruit is unavailable, you can substitute rehydrated dried fruit such as unsulfured apricots, prunes, or figs. For directions on how to make nut butter and rehydrate dried fruit, see Appendix A.

For the starch, make your selection from the "Suggested Starches" on page 194. If you elect to have a whole-grain cereal, use as little heat as possible to properly cook it. Preferably, cook the cereal in a double boiler or thermos. For directions on cooking cereal in a thermos, see "Thermos Cooking" on page 195. For your beverage, make your selection from the "Suggested Beverages" on page 196.

In addition to the fruit, starch, and healthy beverage, you should have one or more of the following supplements—sunflower-seed meal, rice polishings, wheat germ, flaxseed meal, dulse powder, or vegetable-broth powder. Sprinkle about a teaspoon of each of your selected supplements on your cereal or fruit.

To see how easy it is to put together a healthy and delicious breakfast, see the following suggested breakfast menus. Note that fourteen menus are offered for breakfast, as opposed to the seven each that are given for lunch and dinner, to show how much variety is possible. Many people have the most difficulty planning this important first meal of the day.

Suggested Starches

The following starches are particularly good for use on the
Health and Harmony Food Regimen:

❑ Banana and Hubbard squashes

❑ Bananas, raw or baked (when eaten raw, bananas should
  be very ripe)

❑ Barley

❑ Bran muffins

❑ Brown rice, steamed

❑ Cooked cereals such as millet, steel-cut oatmeal, and
  whole-wheat

❑ Crisp rye wafers

❑ Potatoes, baked

❑ Whole-wheat, multiple-grain, corn, or soybean bread

❑ Wild rice, steamed

  See the menu plans for additional starches to consume
as part of this dietary regimen.

Day One

Rehydrated dried apricots
Steel-cut oatmeal
Oat straw tea (see page 197)
Selected supplements (sunflower-seed meal, rice polishings, wheat
germ, flaxseed meal, dulse powder, and/or vegetable-broth powder)
Soft-boiled or poached eggs (optional)

Day Two

Sliced peaches
Cottage cheese
Herbal tea
Selected supplements

Thermos Cooking

You can prepare cooked cereal without spending precious time in the kitchen when you have to hurry off to work or school. The night before, simply pour your uncooked cereal into a wide-mouthed vacuum bottle. Add enough boiling water to create the consistency desired and seal the bottle. That's it! By morning, your cereal will be cooked and ready to eat.

Thermos cooking is not only convenient, but avoids the use of nutrition-robbing high heat. Another bonus is that you can steer clear of those expensive, nutritionally deficient, processed instant cereals. Thermos cooking is a great way to take hot cereal in the car when you go on a trip. It's also terrific when camping, since it uses no hard-to-clean pots or pans.

Day Three

Fresh figs
Cornmeal cereal
Shave grass tea
Selected supplements
Eggs, any style, or nut butter (optional)

Day Four

Raw applesauce and blackberries
Coddled or poached eggs
Herbal tea
Selected supplements

Day Five

Rehydrated dried peaches
Millet cereal
Alfalfa-mint tea
Selected supplements
Eggs, any style, cheese, or nut butter (optional)

Suggested Beverages

The following beverages are particularly good for use on the Health and Harmony Food Regimen:

❑ Alfalfa-mint tea

❑ Buttermilk

❑ Coffee substitute

❑ Dr. Jensen's Favorite Health Drink (see page 202 for the recipe)

❑ Huckleberry tea

❑ Oat straw tea (see page 197 for the recipe)

❑ Papaya tea

❑ Raw milk

❑ Soups such as carrot, leek, cream of celery, and cream of lentil soup

❑ Vegetable broth

See the menu plans for additional beverages to consume as part of this dietary regimen.

Day Six

Sliced nectarines and apple
Plain unsweetened yogurt
Herbal tea
Selected supplements

Day Seven

Prunes and any rehydrated dried fruit
Brown rice
Oat straw tea
Selected supplements

Oat Straw Tea

Oat straw tea is recommended for use on the Health and Harmony Food Regimen because of its high silicon content. Silicon is a mineral directly associated with the health of the skin, hair, and nails. If you look closely at oat straw, you will see that the stalk has a shiny, smooth outer covering. Its appearance stems from its silicon content. When the body lacks silicon, the hair loses its luster, becomes brittle, and falls out more easily. Nails become brittle and crack, and the skin becomes wrinkled and dry from loss of elasticity.

To make oat straw tea, use one heaping teaspoon of chopped loose oat straw in approximately one and one-quarter cups of water. Bring the mixture to a rolling boil and allow it to boil vigorously for at least ten minutes in order to leach the silicon from the straw. Mere steeping is not sufficient. Be very watchful, as this tea tends to boil over very quickly. Strain the mixture and drink the tea warm.

Oat straw is also known as horsetail. Oat straw tea is very mild and has a pleasant, delicate flavor. Add a little honey to it, if desired. You may use oat straw tea as frequently as you wish.

Day Eight

Grapefruit and kumquats
Poached eggs
Herbal tea
Selected supplements

Day Nine

Sliced fresh pineapple with shredded coconut
Buckwheat cereal
Peppermint tea
Selected supplements

Day Ten

Baked apple or stewed persimmons
Chopped raw almonds
Acidophilus milk
Herbal tea
Selected supplements

Day Eleven

Muesli with added sliced bananas and dates
Raw milk
Dandelion coffee or herbal tea
Selected supplements

Day Twelve

Raw applesauce with raisins
Rye cereal
Shave grass tea
Selected supplements

Day Thirteen

Sliced cantaloupe and strawberries
Cottage cheese
Herbal tea
Selected supplements

Day Fourteen

Sliced banana and strawberries
Steel-cut oatmeal
Herbal tea
Selected supplements
Eggs, any style, or nut butter (optional)

Mid-Morning Snack

At 10:30 A.M., you may have a mid-morning snack. An excellent morning snack is vegetable broth or a six- to eight-ounce glass of vegetable juice or fruit juice. Both broth and juice are healthy and will blunt your hunger, but will not make you too full to enjoy a nutritious lunch around noon.

Lunch

Lunch should consist of a raw salad, one or two starches, and a healthy beverage. To make the salad, mix together four or five items from the "Suggested Salad Vegetables" on page 200. Select your starches from the "Suggested Starches" on page 194, and your beverage from the "Suggested Beverages" on page 196.

You may have your noon meal in place of your evening meal, but if you do, you must still follow your same daily routine. It takes exercise to properly digest raw food, and we generally get more exercise after the noon meal. This is why I advise having raw salad at noon.

To show you how easy it is plan a healthy and tasty lunch, I have put together seven suggested menus as samples.

Day One

Raw salad
Baby lima beans
Baked potato
Spearmint tea

Day Two

Raw salad with healthy mayonnaise such as Hain or Nasoya
Steamed asparagus
Very ripe bananas or steamed unpolished rice
Vegetable broth or herbal tea

Day Three

Raw salad with sour-cream dressing
Cooked green beans and/or baked Hubbard squash
Cornbread
Sassafras tea

Day Four

Raw salad with French dressing
Baked zucchini and okra
Corn on the cob
Crisp rye wafers
Buttermilk or herbal tea

Suggested
Salad Vegetables

The following vegetables are particularly good for use in raw salads on the Health and Harmony Food Regimen:

- ❏ Alfalfa sprouts
- ❏ Asparagus
- ❏ Avocado
- ❏ Bean sprouts
- ❏ Carrots
- ❏ Celery
- ❏ Cucumber

- ❏ Green peppers
- ❏ Okra
- ❏ Onions
- ❏ Pimentos
- ❏ Radishes
- ❏ Turnips
- ❏ Zucchini

To make a raw salad, mix four or five of the above vegetables with plenty of the following:

- ❏ Greens such as watercress, spinach, beet leaves, parsley, endive, young chard, herbs, and cabbage
- ❏ Lettuce such as romaine, Boston, and red leaf
- ❏ Tomatoes

If you wish, add a healthy dressing to the salad.

Day Five

Raw salad
Baked green pepper stuffed with sliced eggplant and tomatoes
Baked potato and/or bran muffin
Carrot soup or herbal tea

Day Six

Raw salad
Steamed turnips and turnip greens

Baked yam
Catnip tea

Day Seven

Raw salad with lemon and olive oil
Steamed whole barley
Cream of celery soup
Steamed chard
Herbal tea

Mid-Afternoon Snack

At 3:00 P.M., you may have a mid-afternoon snack. An excellent after-noon snack is a glass of Dr. Jensen's Favorite Health Drink, a six- to eight-ounce glass of vegetable juice or fruit juice, or a piece of fruit. For the recipe that my wife uses to make my health beverage, see "Dr. Jensen's Favorite Health Drink" on page 202.

Dinner

For dinner, you should have a small raw salad, two cooked vegeta-bles, one protein, and, if desired, a beverage. When making the salad, choose the ingredients from the "Suggested Salad Vegetables" on page 200. Choose your hot vegetables from the "Suggested Cooked Vegetables" on page 203, and your beverage from the "Suggested Beverages" on page 196. If you wish, you may also have a hot or cold soup with dinner.

Once a week, eat a white fish such as sole, halibut, freshwater trout, or sea trout for dinner. Vegetarians may substitute soybeans, lima beans, cottage cheese, sunflower or other seeds, seed butter, nut butter, a nut-milk drink, or eggs. (For directions on how make nut and seed butters, see Appendix A.) An egg omelet is acceptable. Twice a week, you should have cottage cheese or any aged cheese that breaks easily. Three times a week, you may have meat. Always choose a lean meat, and avoid pork, smoked meats, and cured meats. Vegetarians may also use meat substitutes and vegetarian proteins.

On the nights that you have a protein for dinner, remember Die-tary Law Number Nine: the Law of Food Combining. According to this law, certain proteins and starches should not be eaten together. For a full discussion of this dietary law, see page 181. Notice how I keep protein and starch separated in my seven suggested dinner menus.

Dr. Jensen's Favorite Health Drink

This health drink has become a favorite of mine over the years. Whenever I ask my wife, Marie, to prepare "my drink," this is the recipe she uses. This drink serves as a nice pick-me-up in mid-afternoon. It is healthy and delicious. I also use it as a substitute lunch at those times when I am so involved in my work that I don't want to take the time to eat a regular meal.

8 ounces fruit juice, vegetable juice, soymilk, or vegetable broth
¼ avocado
1 tablespoon finely ground hulled sesame seeds or sesame butter
1 teaspoon honey

1. Place all the ingredients in a blender, cover, and blend for one-half minute.

2. Pour into a tall glass and serve.

Day One

Small raw salad
Diced celery and carrots
Steamed spinach
Egg omelet
Vegetable broth

Day Two

Small raw salad
Cooked beet tops
Broiled beef such as steak or prime ribs
Cauliflower
Comfrey tea

Suggested
Cooked Vegetables

The following cooked vegetables are particularly good for
use on the Health and Harmony Food Regimen:

❑ Artichokes   ❑ Onions

❑ Beet Tops   ❑ Peas

❑ Beets   ❑ Spinach

❑ Broccoli   ❑ Sprouts

❑ Cabbage   ❑ String beans

❑ Carrots   ❑ Swiss chard

❑ Cauliflower   ❑ Turnips

❑ Eggplant   ❑ Zucchini

In addition to the above vegetables, any vegetable other
than potatoes may be cooked and eaten.

Day Three

Small raw salad
Cottage cheese
Cheese sticks
Apples, peaches, grapes, or a nut butter
  (choose at least two)
Apple juice

Day Four

Small raw salad
Steamed chard
Baked eggplant
Grilled liver and onions
Persimmons
Alfalfa-mint tea

Day Five

Small raw salad with yogurt and lemon
Steamed mixed greens
Beets
Steamed fish with lemon wedge
Leek soup

Day Six

Small raw salad
Cooked string beans
Baked summer squash
Lentil-Carrot Loaf (see page 205 for the recipe)
Cream of lentil soup
Fresh peach gelatin with almond nut cream

Day Seven

Small raw salad
Steamed diced carrots and peas
Tomato aspic
Roast leg of lamb
Mint sauce

IT'S NOT JUST WHAT YOU EAT THAT COUNTS, BUT ALSO WHAT YOU ABSORB

We have seen that in any attempt to manage the bowel, diet must be taken into consideration. If you do not do this, you may become a "doctor shopper," running from one doctor to the next in search of better health while your disease condition becomes ever more chronic because you aren't dealing with the cause.

Diet is important in gaining and maintaining health, but there is another factor besides the content of the diet that is vital. Even though you may eat the correct foods, you may not always get the maximum benefit from them. The body can utilize only what it is able to absorb.

When considering dietary changes during disease stages, you must also consider your digestive ability. For instance, a colitis patient cannot eat a big raw salad right off the bat, even though raw salads are wonderful. In a colitis patient, the bowel wall is in no condition to handle such roughage. The bowel must first be soothed, then cleansed, and finally built up enough to be able to digest these foods.

Lentil-Carrot Loaf

Lentil-Carrot Loaf not only makes an excellent meal, but is a wonderful company dish when served on a platter surrounded by sliced ripe tomatoes, sliced radishes, or any other colorful vegetable.

3 cups (⅓-inch-thick) carrot slices
1½ cups cooked and drained lentils
1 cup rolled oats
½ cup finely chopped onions
2 tablespoons finely chopped parsley
2 tablespoons tamari

1. Preheat the oven to 350°F. Oil a loaf pan.

2. Steam and drain the carrots. Place in a large bowl.

3. Add the lentils to the carrots and mash with a potato masher. Add the remaining ingredients and mix well. Pour into the loaf pan and bake for thirty-five to forty minutes.

4. Remove the loaf from the oven and let stand for five minutes. To serve, turn out onto a platter and slice.

Once the bowel's ability to absorb has begun improving, the diet can be gradually increased in coarseness and fiber content. At first, however, broths and light soups are best. After that should come steamed and puréed vegetables and fruits. You can enjoy that nice big raw salad when the bowel is able to handle more bulk, but you should at first consume it in the form of a liquid salad—that is, a salad liquefied in a blender so that it can be digested easily without taxing the intestines. (For complete directions on how to make a liquid salad, see Appendix A.) As your bowel becomes healthier and stronger, you can expand your diet to include foods closer and closer to their natural forms.

THE ROAD TO HEALTHFUL LIVING

By now, I am sure you are aware of the relationship between bowel health and overall physical health. The relationship is a two-way street—you cannot be healthy if your bowel is not functioning at its optimum, and your bowel cannot be healthy if you are not living healthfully. The following "rules" will help you to achieve maximum physical—and spiritual—well-being:

❑ If your last meal has not left you entirely comfortable in mind and body, skip the next meal.

❑ Eat only if you have a keen desire for the plainest food.

❑ Do not eat beyond your needs. Do not eat to satiety.

❑ Be sure to thoroughly chew your food.

❑ Forego a meal if you are in pain, emotionally upset, not hungry, chilled, or overheated.

❑ Never eat during acute illness.

❑ Skin brush daily.

❑ Use a slant board daily.

❑ Exercise daily.

❑ Sniff breathe daily.

❑ Do not smoke or drink alcohol.

❑ Go to bed early. If you are sick, rest more than normal. Work out any problems in the morning; don't take them to bed with you. Sleep with good ventilation to the outdoors.

I hope you understand that managing the bowel requires caution and great care. We must use what is known as common sense, while remembering Voltaire's remark that "common sense is not so common." Remember, too, that some digestive conditions require more than common sense. In such cases, you will need the experience and knowledge of a health professional to guide you. Don't ever be afraid to seek counsel.

Conclusion

Should the body sue the mind before a court of judicature for damages, it would be found that the mind had been a ruinous tenant to its landlord.

—Essays of Plutarch

I have devoted my energies to discovering the secrets of a happy, healthy, long life. Searching the world over for examples of these blessings has been quite an experience, and one from which I've learned a great deal.

During more than sixty years as a nutritionist trying to help people get and stay well, I've come to one certain conclusion. The number-one symptom, the one that occurs most often in the people I see, is bowel disturbance. The people in most Western societies and cultures suffer from digestive or elimination malfunctions of some kind. Gastrointestinal problems are of epidemic proportions. Our food and lifestyle are slowly doing us in by undermining the health and vitality of our great people. Sickness and disease are claiming an ever-greater portion of our energy, time, and money, resulting in increased emotional stress. We are becoming health-poor and vitality-bereft. We have strayed from the right path and have been led to a dead end prematurely. This is unfortunate, but not inescapable. By turning around and giving up the old, by cleansing and taking the higher path, we can once again enjoy the wonderful blessings of a healthy, vital life just as the Creator intended.

We must defy modern society's life-robbing habits and foods by refusing to partake of them anymore. We must be willing to cut loose from the old and be like a little child once again, learning new and better ways. Surgery and medications merely delay or suppress problems, rarely, if ever, reaching the sources of our diseases. This is why it is said that one operation leads to another. Medications are given to alleviate symptoms, and they often mask deeper and more chronic conditions that go undetected and uncared for until, often, they are too advanced to be corrected.

There is one sure way to deal with our health problems. That one way is God's way. To say "God's way" is the same as saying "nature's way." When we follow nature, we can't lose. God is our Father, but nature is our mother. We are created by God, the Father, and sustained by nature, the mother. Like God, Mother Nature always works to promote health and sustain life. Ultimately, nature is beyond man's tampering and contains all the preconditions for a long and healthy life.

It takes a long time to develop a chronic, degenerative disease, and it takes a long time to reverse such a condition. I believe disease reversal is possible if the individual can commit himself or herself to the task and adhere to nature's ways. I've worked in bowel management all my life. I've tried nearly every natural method, product, and technique known to man that is supposed to be beneficial to the bowel. I have concluded that the Ultimate Tissue Cleansing Program is the greatest thing I've ever found to detoxify the body and clean the bowel. This is a relatively recent development in my life, but one I had been working for and anticipating for a long time. Luckily, it arrived just when we needed it more than ever. I'm not saying it's a cure-all, but it is a very powerful beginning for a person who is working toward an eventual healing.

Anything we can do to stop autointoxication will help slow down the disease process. The Ultimate Tissue Cleansing Program is the best way I know to accomplish this goal. By stripping down the old, toxic mucous lining of the bowel, we remove the number-one source of disease in the body. In addition, we open up the bowel to a more efficient means of waste elimination and nutrient absorption, both of which are essential to any lasting healing process. This is also the first step toward normalizing the bowel so that the friendly bacteria will return to keep the colon safe from putrefaction and further autointoxication.

Consider the following story told by J. Oswold Empringham in his book *Pandora's Box: What to Eat and Why*. The story is about one of the longest-lived men in Western history:

Westminster Abbey was begun by King Lucius in 170 A.D. The vaults are crowded with illustrious dead whose monuments cover the floor and walls of that vast church. One of the smallest slabs—more interesting than all the fine marbles to princes and poets says:

"Thomas Parr of ye county of Salopp, born A.D. 1483. He lived in ye reigns of ten kings: Edward IV, Edward V, Richard III, Henry VII, Henry VIII, Edward VI, Mary, Elizabeth, James I, Charles I. Buried here November 15, 1635. Aged 152 years."

Before Parr was interred in Westminster, his history was carefully investigated. The parish register of his native village proves he was baptized in 1483. Legal documents and court entries show that he inherited a small farm from his father in 1560, and that he took a wife three years later when 80. He married again in 1605 at the age of 122. When over 130, he pleaded guilty, in court, to the charge of fathering an illegitimate child. He was a farmer all his life. His great age attracted the notice of the King who invited him to the palace for a visit, as the King wished to investigate his exceptional longevity. Parr's last days were spent in the palace. History says his perfect faculties and marvelous memory made him a matchless entertainer. No wonder. What reminiscences a man who had lived ten reigns must have had!

After Parr's death, William Harvey, the English physiologist who discovered the circulation of the blood, performed an autopsy, by order of King Charles, to find out why Parr had lived so long. The great physician's report in Latin, still preserved, states that Parr died from acute indigestion brought on by indulgences in unaccustomed luxuries. All of the old man's organs were in perfect condition, and Harvey describes the colon as normal in position and in other respects like that of a child. Modern microbiologists say that in this report, Harvey unknowingly reveals the secret of Parr's long life, because his minute description of the intestines proves that the congenital, protective flora had not been lost.

Let Parr's secret help you choose the level of consciousness on which you live. The Muscular Dystrophy campaign's phrase "Your Change is the Key to the Cure" has more portent than we realize. I would like you to take a look at the negative aspects of your life and answer the question, "What are these to you?" Then I would like to hand you a pair of imaginary scissors and have you to cut these negative aspects off, so you can be free of them, lose them, let them go. There are some things in life that are not good for us, and we need to cut them loose.

"He leadeth me beside still waters." Do you know where the stillness is? Get rid of the confusion and mental chatter that you've had in the past. "Be still, and know." Take a little time to find out who you are and where you are going. Go forward with a sign on your back that says, "Under New Management!" When you can do this, you will be able to meet the new day with a refreshed spirit. As you are able to do this, your healing will come.

Photographs

Warning: The following photographs are very graphic. Sensitive individuals may not wish to view them.

The photographs on the following pages show the kinds of results I have obtained from the Ultimate Tissue Cleansing Program. If a photograph was ever worth a thousand words, these surely are. I have never experienced any other tissue-cleansing method with results as consistent and thorough as this one. These photographs show that the Ultimate Tissue Cleansing Program is truly a major step forward in the battle to overcome toxemia and autointoxication.

On pages 213 to 215 are a photographic record of how the Ultimate Tissue Cleansing Program reversed a stubborn case of ulcerated feet and ankles. The pages each focus on a different view of the feet, but on each of the pages, the first photo was taken on Day One of the treatment, the second photo on Day Four, and the third photo on Day Seven. The results of the cleanse were remarkable.

On pages 216 to 220 are photographs showing the putrefactive debris that came from twenty-eight different individuals who undertook the seven-day cleanse. Who would ever guess that such things could accumulate inside the human body? Could this substance be the source of disease, illness, and poor health? The material shown ranges from jelly-like to as hard as truck-tire rubber, from clear to as black as tar, from fresh to morbidly old, and from fragments to four-foot-long ropes, all with odors that speak only of very rotten things. Notice how the mucous lining, when firm enough, took the shape of the bowel, complete with haustrations, striations, strictures, and diverticula. This is truly an amazing phenomenon.

Pages 221 to 222 clearly illustrate Hering's Law of Cure. Here we can see the results of tissue cleansing combined with proper nutition. This insulin-dependent diabetic was able to maintain a lower blood-sugar level for the duration of the program using much less insulin than he normally required. The patient's medical history included psoriasis for seven years, diabetes for four years, and arthritis for two years. As the photos show, his symptoms retreated in the reverse order of their arrival. This series of photographs is visual proof of Hering's wonderful law.

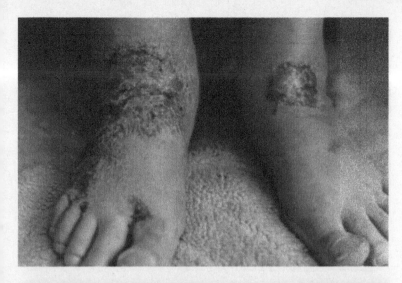

DAY 1

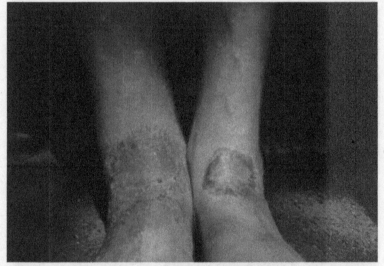

DAY 4

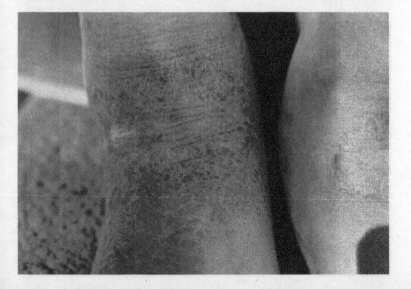

DAY 7

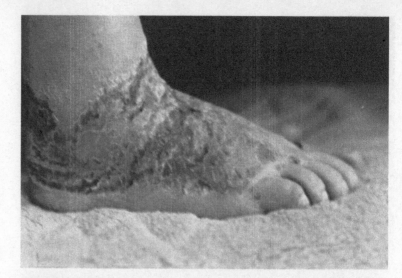

DAY 1

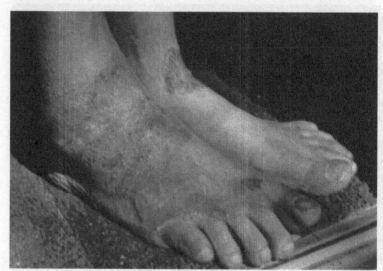

DAY 4

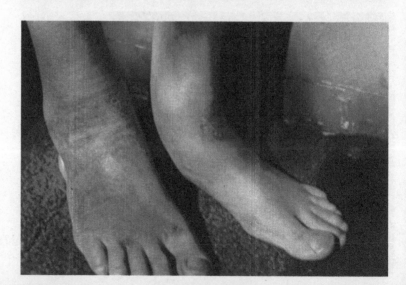

DAY 7

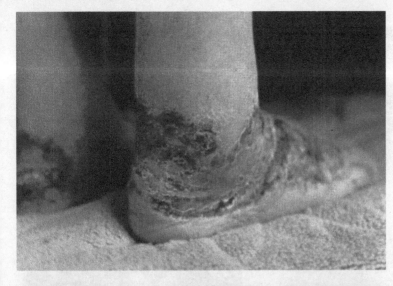

DAY 1

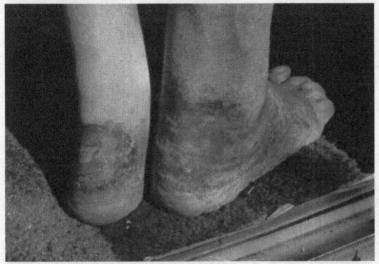

DAY 4

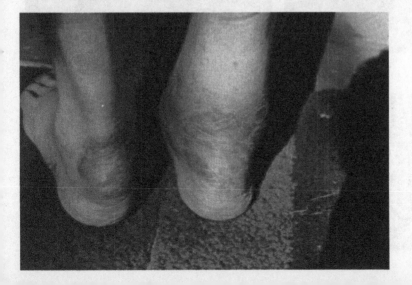

DAY 7

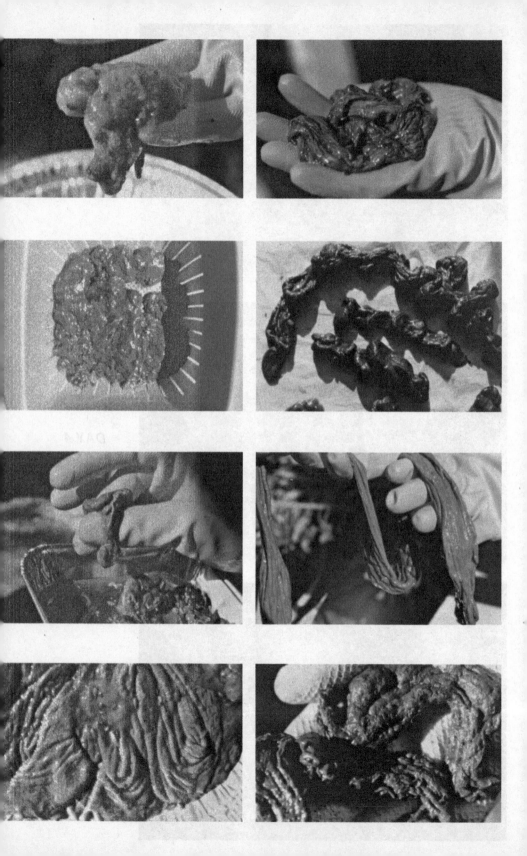

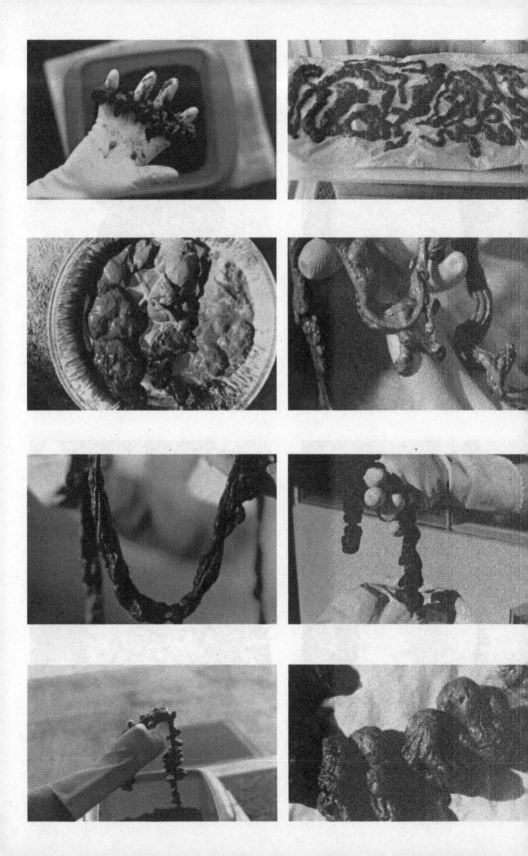

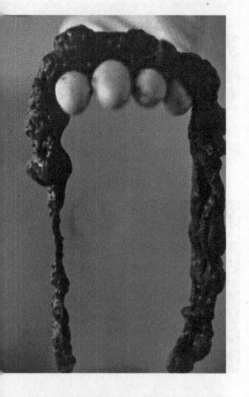
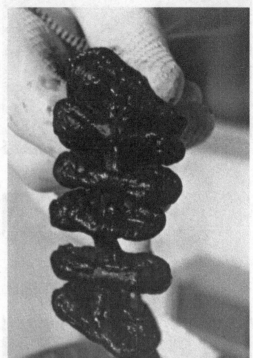
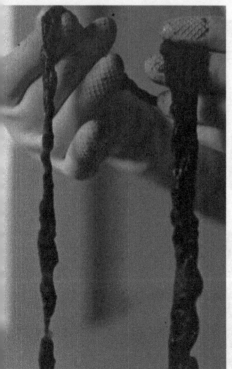
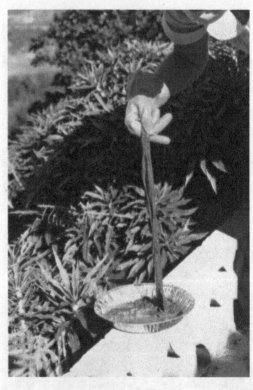

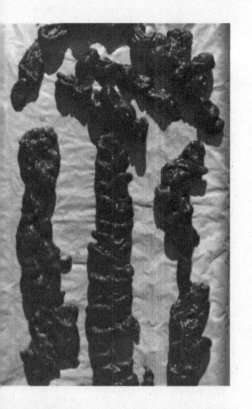
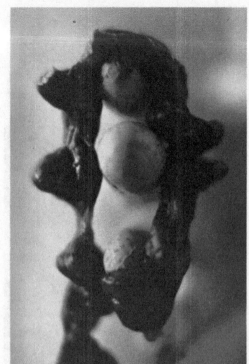
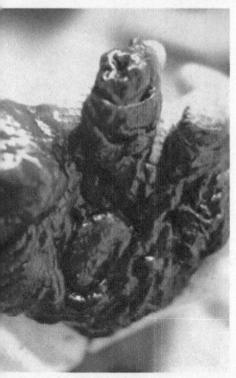
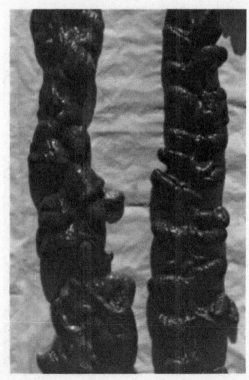

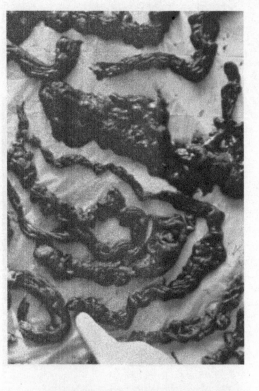
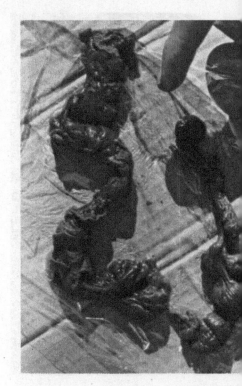
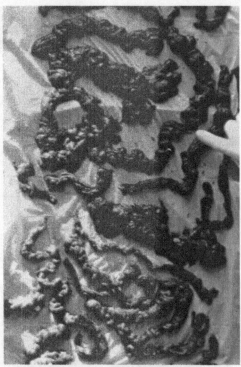
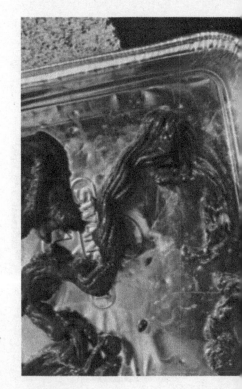

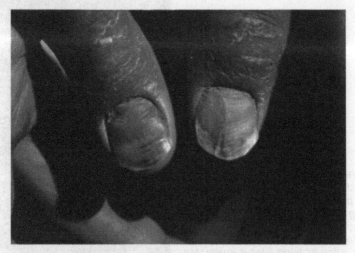

PAINFUL PSORIASIS IN ACUTE STAGE

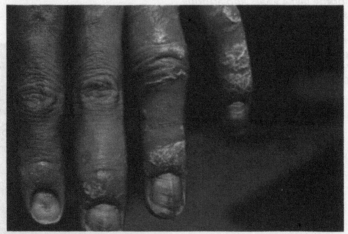

SYMPTOMS RETREAT FOLLOWING TISSUE CLEANSING TREATMENT

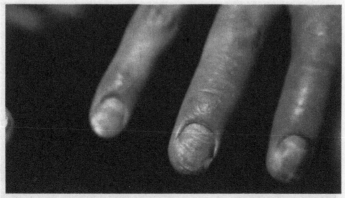

HEALING AND REJUVENATION FOLLOWING DETOXIFICATION

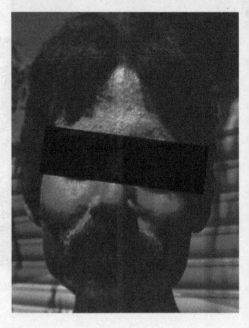

Hering's law of cure is clearly illustrated in the following photographs. Here we can see the results of the tissue cleansing treatment as it is combined with good nutritional support. This insulin-dependent diabetic was able to maintain a lower-level blood sugar for the extent of the tissue toxin elimination diet with much less insulin. This patient has had psoriasis for the last 7 years, diabetes for the last 4 years and arthritis for the last 2 years. As you can see, the psoriasis is leaving, as are all the other symptoms. The most recent afflictions are leaving more quickly while the older ones are retreating more slowly, as in the "reverse order."

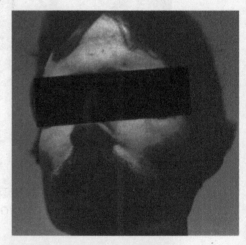

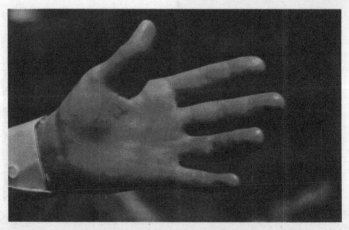

Appendix A

Directions for Preparing Special Foods

Several special foods are used on the Ultimate Tissue Cleansing Program and the Health and Harmony Food Regimen. Following are the simplest ways I have found to make these foods.

REHYDRATED DRIED FRUIT

Dried fruit is very good because it can be kept for an extended period. Dried foods also take up very little storage space and can be used when fresh foods are unavailable. However, I do not recommend that you consume fruit in its dried form. Try to find fresh fruit, but if none is available, rehydrated dried fruit is an acceptable substitute.

The best way to rehydrate dried fruit is to place it in a saucepan with cold water and let it soak for a while. Then, slowly bring the fruit and water to the boiling point, reduce the heat, and let the fruit simmer for two minutes. Remove the saucepan from the heat, cover, and let the fruit and water cool overnight. In the morning, the fruit will be plumped up and ready to eat. This process not only rehydrates the fruit, but destroys any eggs and germs that may be on the fruit.

When shopping for dried or fresh fruit look for organically grown fruit. This kind of fruit is best for making juice. To cook fruit, waterless cookware with a lid that forms a vapor seal is best.

NUT AND SEED BUTTERS

Any edible nuts or seeds—except sesame seeds—can be used to make a nut or seed butter. Because of their small size, sesame seeds pass through the grinding teeth of food processors without being masticated. You can purchase sesame-seed butter, and many other nut and seed butters, in health-food stores. Sesame seeds are also available as a purée called tahini, and as a mash formed into bars or cakes known as halvah.

When preparing your own butters, remember that some nuts, such as walnuts, have very little oil content and therefore do not purée well unless a measure of oil is added as the nuts are processed. Cashews also process better with a little added oil. Safflower oil is preferable because its flavor is very mild and doesn't alter the taste of the nuts. You can make peanut butter, too, but peanuts are a legume, not a nut, and are not as digestible as most nut and seed butters.

All nut and seed butters must be refrigerated, as they will become rancid if stored at room temperature. Nut and seed butters are excellent eaten plain, on crackers and bread, and with salads and fruit.

Do not eat nuts and seeds unless they are in butter form. Most people do not chew nuts and seeds well enough, and the small chunks may lodge in diverticula.

LIQUID SALAD

People who have digestive problems or cannot chew well often benefit from consuming their salads in liquid form. Greens and other raw salad materials, though excellent sources of fiber, can irritate the digestive tract of people who have inflammations or are sensitive to a lot of roughage. Most of these people can instead consume their salads in liquid form, as a drink.

To make a liquid salad, simply place the salad materials in a high-speed blender, add water, and liquefy. Greens, especially when fractionated, tend to have a bitter taste because of their potassium content. To offset this taste, I usually add some carrot juice.

Appendix B

Where to Find Special Products

Most of the items needed to complete the Ultimate Tissue Cleansing Program are available in health-food and other stores. However, several pieces of the necessary equipment may need to be purchased by mail.

COLEMA BOARDS AND BUCKETS

Colema boards are made by several commercial producers. I use a board made by Ultimate Trends, Inc., because of its size and easy cleaning. All the boards currently available are worth investigating, however. If you send for information, you will receive diagrams showing how the boards are set up, shipping instructions, and directions for using the boards when traveling. You can also find out which models are designed for comfort, which ones are best for heavier people, and so on. The Ultimate Trends board is made by Eldon L. Lowd, 7835 South 1300 East, Sandy, UT 84092. A folding board is manufactured by Colema Boards of California, Inc., and is available through Bernard Jensen International, 24360 Old Wagon Road, Escondido, CA 92027, and Dr. Donald Bodeen, 219 New Hackensack Road, Poughkeepsie, NY 12603. In western Canada, colema boards can be obtained through Lenard Moodie, 45 Doverville Way, S.E., Calgary, AB T2B 2N6.

All colema boards come complete with the necessary tubing and other attachments, as well as two rectal tips. Buckets are not included with every board, but can be requested. Any clean, strong four- to five-gallon bucket can be used for colemas. I obtain food-grade plastic buckets with lids from a local restaurant-supply house and add my own spigot. I recommend you obtain your bucket locally, since buckets are inexpensive and cost almost as much to ship as to purchase.

COLEMA SUPPLIES

All of the supplies needed for the Ultimate Tissue Cleansing Program are available through Bernard Jensen International, 24360 Old Wagon Road, Escondido, CA 92027, and Dr. Donald Bodeen, 219 New Hackensack Road, Poughkeepsie, NY 12603. Most of the items are also available at appropriate retail outlets, such as health-food stores, pharmacies, and hardware stores.

SLANT BOARDS

Slant boards can be purchased at most stores that sell exercise or gym equipment. Sears has also carried slant boards. Folding slant boards that have carrying handles and can be easily transported and stored are manufactured by the York Barbell Company, Box 1707, York, PA 17405. They are available through Bernard Jensen International, 24360 Old Wagon Road, Escondido, CA 92027, and Dr. Donald Bodeen, 219 New Hackensack Road, Poughkeepsie, NY 12603. Slant boards can also be obtained from Ultimate Trends, Inc, 7835 South 1300 East, Sandy, UT 84092, and Jennings Home Colonic Boards, P.O. Box 1495, Anderson, CA 96007. In Canada, they can be obtained from Take Care Health Products, Box 538, 1755 Robson Street, Vancouver, BC V6G 1C9.

If you make your own slant board, make sure that it is wide enough to support your body. It should also be longer than you are tall so that your head rests on the board, not on the floor. One end of the board should be raised fifteen to eighteen inches above the floor. Make sure that the elevated end is well supported to prevent accidents and injuries. Add ankle straps at the foot end to keep your body from sliding down the board and to provide gravity-induced traction on the spine.

SKIN BRUSHES

To obtain a long-handled natural-bristle brush perfect for skin brushing, write to Bernard Jensen International, 24360 Old Wagon Road, Escondido, CA 92027, or Dr. Donald Bodeen, 219 New Hackensack Road, Poughkeepsie, NY 12603.

TOILET FOOTSTOOL

To obtain the toilet footstool described on page 151, contact Welles Enterprises, 6565 Balboa Avenue, Suite A, San Diego, CA 92111.

TISSUE-CLEANSING PROGRAMS AND SEMINARS

For information on tissue-cleansing programs and educational seminars, contact Bernard Jensen International, 24360 Old Wagon Road, Escondido, CA 92027, or Dr. Donald Bodeen, 219 New Hackensack Road, Poughkeepsie, NY 12603.

Glossary

The italicized words are defined elsewhere in the glossary.

acidophilus. A friendly *lactobacillus* bacteria normally in the colon.

adhesion. A holding-together of two normally separate structures by new tissue that was produced because of inflammation or injury.

adsorbent. Capable of assimilating matter onto its surface.

albumin. A protein found in nearly every animal tissue and many vegetable tissues, and characterized by water solubility and heat coagulability.

anus. The outlet of the *rectum* lying in the fold between the buttocks.

arteriosclerosis. Hardening of the arteries.

ascending colon. The part of the colon that rises up from the *cecum* to the *hepatic flexure*.

atherosclerosis. A condition in which fatty-type materials accumulate on the walls of the arteries.

autointoxication. A condition caused by poisonous substances produced within the body.

bursa. Body cavities, particularly between joints.

bursitis. An inflammation of a *bursa*, especially in the shoulder, elbow, or knee.

catarrh. An inflammation of the *mucous membranes*.

cecum. The dilated intestinal pouch into which the *ileum*, *ascending colon*, and appendix open.

celiac disease. A condition of intestinal *malabsorption* characterized by *diarrhea*, malnutrition, a tendency to bleed, and reduced calcium in the blood.

229

chyme. The mixture of partly digested food and digestive secretions that moves through the small intestine during digestion.

cold pressed. A meaningless term referring to the process in which oil is extracted from seeds. Oils cannot be commercially pressed cold. The usual temperatures reach about 100°C (212°F). The term was coined by the oil manufacturers for advertising purposes.

colloidal suspension. A liquid in which such fine particles are suspended that they do not separate out. The cream or fat in homogenized milk is an example of a colloid.

colonic. Pertaining to the colon. Also, a means of washing out the colon using a device that allows water to flow into and out of the colon to carry out waste material.

colostomy. A surgically constructed excretory opening from the colon.

constipation. Difficult defecation; infrequent defecation, with passage of unduly hard and dry fecal material; sluggish action of the bowels.

cyanosis. A bluish discoloration of the skin resulting from inadequate oxygenation of the blood.

decoction. A tea made from the bark, roots, seeds, or berries of a plant. Instead of being steeped, however, most herbs are simmered for about twenty to thirty minutes.

descending colon. The part of the colon that travels downward from the *splenic flexure* to the sigmoid colon.

diarrhea. The frequent passage of watery bowel movements. It is often a symptom of gastrointestinal disturbances and is primarily the result of increased *peristalsis*.

diverticula. The plural of *diverticulum*.

diverticulitis. An inflammation of one or more *diverticula* in the intestinal tract, especially in the colon, caused by trapped feces.

diverticulosis. The presence of diverticula, particularly in the intestines.

diverticulum. A sac or pouch in the wall of a canal or organ.

duodenum. The first portion of the small intestine, extending from the *pylorus* to the *jejunum*.

eclampsia. A condition of convulsions and coma occurring in pregnant women and new mothers. It is associated with elevated blood pressure, water retention, and protein in the urine; it rarely involves coma alone. Eclampsia is a medical emergency.

edema. A swelling of tissue, often associated with water retention.

electrolyte. An ion required by the body to regulate the electric charge and flow of water between the cells and the bloodstream. The primary electrolytes are sodium, potassium, and chloride.

electrolyte balance. The ratio of sodium, potassium, chloride, and the other *electrolytes* in the body.

enema. A method of introducing solutions into the *rectum* and colon to stimulate bowel activity and to cause emptying of the lower intestine.

fistula. An abnormal passage or communication, usually between two internal organs, but sometimes from an internal organ to the surface of the body.

flaccid. Relaxed; flabby; having defective or absent muscular tone.

flatulence. Gas in the stomach and intestines.

frozen shoulder. An inflammation and swelling of the shoulder joint with *adhesions* that immobilize the shoulder.

glycogen. A complex carbohydrate that is the storage form of glucose.

haustra. The normal pouches of the colon.

hemorrhoid. Swollen veins located just inside, just outside, or across the walls of the *anus*.

hepatic. Pertaining to the liver.

hepatic flexure. The turn or bend in the part of the colon that is nearest the liver; the bend where the *ascending colon* turns to form the *transverse colon*.

hernia. The protrusion or projection of an organ or a part of an organ through the wall of the cavity that normally contains it.

hydrogenated. The addition of hydrogen to an unsaturated compound, usually a fat. When all the bonding sites are filled with hydrogen, the compound is saturated. When some of the bonding sites are filled, the compound is partially hydrogenated.

hyper-. A prefix meaning "above," "excessive," or "beyond."

hypertension. High blood pressure.

hypo-. A prefix meaning "less than," "below," or "under."

ileocecal valve. The group of *sphincter* muscles that serves to close the *ileum* at the point where the small intestine opens into the *ascending colon*. It prevents food material from re-entering the small intestine.

ileum. The portion of the small intestine that extends from the *jejunum* to the *cecum*.

indican. The potassium salt of indoxylsulfate, found in sweat and urine, and formed when intestinal bacteria convert the amino acid tryptophan into *indole*.

indole. A solid, crystalline substance found in feces. It is the product of the bacterial decomposition of the amino acid tryptophan and is largely responsible for the odor of feces. In intestinal obstruction, it is absorbed and eliminated in the urine as *indican*.

international unit. A measure of potency based on an accepted international standard.

interstitial. Pertaining to a gap or space between tissues or structure parts.

intestinal flora. The bacteria present in the intestine.

intraluminal. Within the cavity of a tube or tubular organ.

IU. The abbreviation of *international unit*.

jejunum. The portion of the small intestine that extends from the *duodenum* to the *ileum*.

lacteal. In this discussion, an intestinal lymphatic vessel that takes up *chyme* and passes it to the *lymph* circulation and, by way of the *thoracic* duct, to the bloodstream.

lactobacillus. Any of the bacteria of the genus *Lactobacillus* that ferment lactic acid from milk sugar. They are natural inhabitants of the colon and are called "friendly bacteria" because they aid in digestion and help fight certain diseases. The most common *lactobacilli* available in supplemental form are *Lactobacillus acidophilus*, *Lactobacillus bifidus*, and *Lactobacillus bulgaricus*.

laxative. A food or chemical substance that acts to loosen the bowels and, therefore, is used to prevent or treat *constipation*. Laxatives act by increasing *peristalsis* by irritating the intestinal *mucosa*, lubricating the intestinal walls, softening the bowel contents by increasing the amount of water in the intestines, or increasing the bulk of the bowel contents.

live foods. Natural foods that have their enzymes, vitamins, and minerals intact; organically grown, unprocessed, raw foods.

lumen. The interior of a tube or tubular organ.

lymph. An alkaline fluid found in the lymphatic vessels. It is usually a clear, transparent, colorless fluid. However, in vessels draining the intestines, it may appear milky owing to the presence of absorbed fats.

lymphocyte. A *lymph* cell or white blood corpuscle without cytoplasmic granules. Lymphocytes normally comprise less than half of the total number of white cells.

lysozyme. An enzyme that has the ability to destroy the cell walls of certain bacteria. Lysozymes are sometimes used as antiseptics.

malabsorption. Incorrect absorption.

malaise. A vague, nonspecific feeling of bodily discomfort.

morbid. Pertaining to or affected by disease. Diseased.

mucilaginous. Have a slimy, sticky texture.

mucosa. *See* mucous membrane.

mucous membrane. One of the membranes lining the cavities and canals of the body that communicate with the air. Included are the membranes lining the inside of the mouth, nose, *anus*, and vagina.

mucus. A thick, sticky fluid secreted by the *mucous membranes* and glands.

muesli. A cold cereal consisting of mixed grains, nuts, and fruit.

myositis. An inflammation of muscle tissue.

norepinephrine. An adrenal hormone that raise the blood pressure by narrowing the blood vessels.

parasite. A plant or animal that lives upon or within another living organism, from whom it obtains some advantage without compensation.

pathological. Of or pertaining to disease.

peristalsis. A progressive, wavelike movement that occurs involuntarily in hollow tubes of the body, especially the digestive system. In the digestive system, it helps move the *chyme* and later the fecal material through the bowel and out the *anus*.

Peyer's patch. An group of *lymph* nodes where the small and large intestine are joined.

photophobia. An extreme intolerance of light.

potable. Fit for drinking.

probiotic. A friendly bacteria that makes conditions in the bowel inhospitable for undesirable bacteria.

prolapsus. A falling or downward displacement of some part of the body, such as the colon or uterus.

proteolytic. Referring to something that breaks proteins into simpler substances.

pyloric. Referring to the *pylorus*.

pylorus. The opening between the stomach and *duodenum*.

rectum. The part of the colon extending from the sigmoid flexure to the *anus*.

roughage. Dietary fiber.

sciatica. A painful condition involving the sciatic nerve.

septicemia. An infection of the whole body caused by the spread of germs via the bloodstream.

spasm. An involuntary sudden movement or convulsive muscular contraction.

spastic. Resembling a *spasm* or convulsion.

sphincter. A ringlike band of muscle fibers that constricts a passage or closes a natural orifice.

splenic flexure. The point near the spleen where the *transverse colon* bends and continues downward as the *descending colon*.

stasis. A stagnation in the normal flow of a fluid such as the blood or urine, or of the intestinal mechanism.

tendinitis. An inflammation of a tendon.

tenosynovitis. An inflammation of a tendon sheath.

thoracic. Pertaining to the chest or thorax of the body.

torticollis. Literally, "turtle neck." Often called "wry neck," it is a state in which the neck muscles are chronically contracted, producing twisting of the neck and an unnatural position of the head.

toxic settlements. Substances, often the residues of drugs, that have settled in inherently weaker tissues of the body.

transverse colon. The section of the colon that travels across the abdomen under the stomach.

Bibliography

Ballentine, Rudolph. *Diet and Nutrition: A Holistic Approach.* Honesdale, PA: Himalayan International Institute, 1979.

Burkitt, Denis P. "Effects of Dietary Fiber on Stools and Transit Times and Its Role in the Causation of Disease." *Lancet* 2 (1972): 1408–1411.

——— and Neil S. Painter. "Dietary Fiber and Disease." *Journal of the American Medical Association* 229 (August 19, 1974):1068–1074.

——— and H.C. Trowell, eds. *Refined Carbohydrate Foods and Disease: Some Implications of Dietary Fiber.* San Diego: Academic Press, 1975.

Clendening, Logan. *The Human Body.* New York: Alfred A. Knopf, 1973.

Empringham, J. Oswald. *Invisible Friends of the Body.* Los Angeles: Health Education Society, n.d.

———. *Pandora's Box: What to Eat and Why.* Los Angeles: Health Education Society, 1970.

The Human Body and How It Works. New York: Exeter Books, 1979.

Jamision, Alcinous B., and Charles A. Tyrrel. *Intestinal Ills.* N.p.: N.p., 1928.

Jensen, Bernard. *Beyond Basic Health.* Garden City Park, NY: Avery Publishing Group, 1988.

———. *Blending Magic.* Escondido, CA: Bernard Jensen Enterprises, 1942.

————. *The Chemistry of Man*. Escondido, CA: Bernard Jensen Enterprises, 1983.

————. *Doctor-Patient Handbook*. Provo, UT: BiWorld, 1976.

————. *Food Healing for Man*. Escondido, CA: Bernard Jensen Enterprises, 1983.

————. *Health Magic Through Chlorophyll From Living Plant Life*. Provo, UT: BiWorld, 1973.

————. *Nature Has a Remedy*. Escondido, CA: Bernard Jensen Enterprises, 1978.

————. *Science and Practice of Iridology*. Provo, UT: BiWorld, 1952.

————. *Survive This Day*. Escondidio, CA: Bernard Jensen Enterprises, 1976.

————. *You Can Master Disease*. Escondido, CA: Bernard Jensen Enterprises, 1976.

———— and Donald V. Bodeen. *Visions of Health*. Garden City Park, NY: Avery Publishing Group, 1992.

Kellog, John Harvey. *Colon Hygiene*. Battle Creek, MI: Good Health Publishing Co., 1923.

Moore, Keith L., and T.V.N. Persaud. *The Developing Human*. Philadelphia: W.B. Saunders, 1973.

Painter, Neil S. *Diverticular Disease of the Colon*. New Canaan, CT: Keats, 1975.

———— and Denis P. Burkitt. "Diverticular Disease of the Colon: A Deficiency Disease of Western Civilization." *British Medical Journal* 2 (1971):450–454.

Schellberg, Boto O. *Lectures on Colonic Therapy*. N.p.: N.p., 1930.

Schmidt, Ray. *Let Food Be Your Medicine and Medicine Your Food*. Hollywood: N.p., n.d.

Szekely, Edmond Bordeaux. *The Essene Gospel of Peace*. Cartago: IBS Internacional, 1978.

Tilden, J.H. *Toxemia: The Basic Cause of Disease*. Chicago: Natural Hygiene Press, 1926.

Trenev, Natasha. *Probiotics*. Garden City Park, NY: Avery Publishing Group, 1998.

Wiltsie, James. *Chronic Intestinal Toxemia and Its Treatment*. N.p.: N.p., 1938.

About the Author

One of America's foremost pioneering nutritionists, Dr. Bernard Jensen began his career in 1929 as a chiropractic physician. He soon turned to the art of nutrition in search of remedies for his own health problems. In his formative years, Dr. Jensen studied under such giants as Dr. Benedict Lust, Dr. John Tilden, Dr. John H. Kellogg, and Dr. V.G. Rocine. Later, he observed firsthand the cultural practices of people in more than fifty-five countries, discovering important links between food and health.

Dr. Jensen has also taught around the world, including in some of the more exotic cities of the Orient. He was invited by the Chinese government to teach iridology on mainland China, and by the Taiwanese to set up a Department of Iridology at a large veterans' hospital in Taipai. He also spent twenty-seven days teaching iridology classes in Malaysia to enthusiastic students. In 1955, Dr. Jensen established the Hidden Valley Ranch in Escondido, California, as a retreat and learning center dedicated to the healing principles of nature.

Over the years, Dr. Jensen has received a multitude of prestigious awards and honors for his work in nutrition and the healing arts. These honors include Knighthood in the Order of St. John of Malta, the Dag Hammarskjold Peace Award of Belgium, and an award from Queen Juliana of the Netherlands. He is also the author of numerous articles and best-selling books. In his nineties, he continues to teach, travel, and learn.

Index